# Insomnia: Psychological Assessment and Management

# TREATMENT MANUALS FOR PRACTITIONERS
David H. Barlow, *Editor*

# Insomnia

Psychological Assessment and Management

CHARLES M. MORIN
Medical College of Virginia
Virginia Commonwealth University

*Series Editor's Note by David H. Barlow*
*Foreword by William C. Dement*

THE GUILFORD PRESS
New York      London

© 1993 The Guilford Press
A Division of Guilford Publications, Inc.
72 Spring Street, New York, NY 10012

Printed in the United States of America

This book is printed on acid-free paper.

Last digit is print number: 9  8  7  6  5  4  3  2

Library of Congress Cataloging-in-Publication Data
Morin, Charles M.
    Insomnia: psychological assessment and management / Charles M. Morin.
       p.    cm.  (Treatment manuals for practitioners)
    Includes bibliographical references and index.
    ISBN 0-89862-210-7.—ISBN 1-57230-120-1 (pbk.)
    1. Insomnia.   I. Title.   II. Series
    [DNLM: 1. Insomnia—therapy.  2. Insomnia—diagnosis.  3. Behavior
Therapy—methods.   WM 188 M858i  1993]
RC548.M67   1993
616.8'498—dc20
DNLM/DLC
for Library of Congress                                    93-6564
                                                               CIP

*To my parents*
*and*
*to a very dear friend, Claude*

# Acknowledgments

This book was written while I was a recipient of a First Independent Research Support and Transition Award (FIRST) from the National Institute of Mental Health (NIMH). Some of the research presented was also supportd by NIMH Grant Nos. 47020 and 44338. The treatment manual is based on clinical practice and research with several hundred insomnia sufferers. I am grateful for all I have learned from these individuals. Some of the procedures presented here were developed and tested by other sleep experts around the world. I am very thankful to these colleagues, from whom I have learned a great deal over the years. I also owe a debt of gratitude to several other people who have contributed to the final product of this book. I am indebted to Dr. Richard Bootzin and Dr. Peter Hauri for their most constructive suggestions on several of the chapters, and to Dr. Doug Brink for his comments on the sleep medication chapter. All staff members of the sleep disorders center at the Medical College of Virginia, as well as students, interns, and fellows, were instrumental in evaluating the efficacy of this treatment protocol. I also wish to thank my secretary, Gwen Johnson, for reading and editing several versions of this book. Finally, I am most grateful to my wife, Paule, for her support and understanding, and for the birth of my daughter, Geneviève, while I was writing this book.

CHARLES M. MORIN

# Series Editor's Note

Perhaps it's our harried existence. Perhaps there is greater recognition of what has been a chronic problem. In any case, disorders of sleep are coming to the forefront of professional concerns and are increasingly more visible in the eyes of the media. One need only refer back to the controversy over the drug Halcion, which has been banned in Britain and is widely held responsible for former President Bush's unfortunate problems in Tokyo, to get some idea of the interest in remedies for disorders of sleep. The negative publicity surrounding Halcion has had a major impact on the profits of one of our large pharmaceutical companies, suggesting how widely it is used.

Advances in our technology have made possible the discovery of substantial amounts of new information concerning sleep and its disorders. The new sleep disorders section in DSM-IV reflects this knowledge in our system of nosology. The increasing interest in these disorders and the growing dissatisfaction with drug remedies among medical and nonmedical professionals alike has once again underscored the importance of developing psychological approaches to sleep disorders. In this volume by Charles Morin, one of the new generation of experts in this area, we have what is probably the most sophisticated nondrug protocol for the treatment of insomnia. Any clinician dealing with sleep disorders, including those who wish to begin to treat these problems in their clinical practice, will find this state-of-the-art clinical program invaluable.

DAVID H. BARLOW
*University at Albany*
*State University of New York*

# Foreword

Our society has arrived at a point in time where it must change the way its institutions and its health professionals deal with sleep. As this book eloquently demonstrates, researchers and practitioners have accumulated an encyclopedic body of knowledge about sleep and the diagnosis and treatment of sleep disorders. However, this knowledge has not diffused into the real world of the home, the schools, the workplace, and community medical practices. Optimal human health and quality of life only exist if sleep is entirely healthy.

With no problem is this more true than insomnia. By far the most common sleep complaint, insomnia affects 20–40% of all adults, especially women and the elderly. However, recent studies by the National Commission on Sleep Disorders Research found that the gatekeepers of medicine, primary care physicians, do not diagnose insomnia. On rare occasions, they offer sleep medication without diagnosis. In the records of more than ten million patients, there was not a single example of an ICD-9 code for a specific insomnia diagnosis.

Most physicians dread the arrival of a patient with severe chronic insomnia. If one asks a large group of physicians if any of them enjoy managing chronic insomnia, not a single hand will go up. The major problem is the sense that nothing can be done, or that achieving a therapeutic improvement is very difficult. Fortunately for medical practitioners, the true insomnia complainer has become a rare event.

In primary care medicine, relatively few patients present with insomnia even as a secondary complaint, let alone primary. It appears that the vast majority of insomniacs have stopped seeking the help of a doctor when they cannot sleep. They are an epidemic of silent sufferers. Apparently, the general public has come to believe (1) that chronic insomnia cannot be helped by physicians except with the administration of sleeping pills which are dangerous, and (2) that insomnia is not really a medical problem.

To the contrary, a recent survey by the National Sleep Foundation found that the complaint of insomnia was associated with very substantial morbidity, with many days lost from work and increased frequency of automobile accidents. Other studies have shown that short sleep is associated with increased mortality.

Current articles and books on insomnia are plentiful, but they either promise too much or do not present clear and effective guidelines for health professionals to respond to such an insomnia complaint or to be proactive and ask in the absence of a complaint.

Dr. Morin's book is a welcome change. In it, he presents us with a clear and well-organized review of the problem of insomnia and a clear and scientifically validated treatment approach. This book can guide the health professional toward an effective and satisfying insomnia practice. It presents a structured and practical approach to the management of insomnia and is "user friendly" for the clinician. We may expect that doctors and other health professionals will begin to feel good about managing insomnia, and confident that they can be successful. We may further hope that word will spread and that people with insomnia will at last get the treatment they deserve.

WILLIAM C. DEMENT, M.D., Ph.D.
*Director, Sleep Disorders Clinic and Research Center
Stanford, University*

*Chairman
National Commission on Sleep Disorders Research*

*Lowell W. and Josephine Q. Berry Professor
of Psychiatry and Behavioral Sciences
Stanford University School of Medicine*

# Preface

This book describes a multifaceted treatment program for chronic insomnia. The manual is divided into three sections. The first section is devoted to assessment and diagnostic issues. After reviewing the nature, prevalence, and impact of insomnia problems, I present some basic facts about sleep and its measurement. The main insomnia subtypes are then described, and diagnostic considerations are discussed. A conceptual model of insomnia is presented, emphasizing the interplay between maladaptive behavior patterns and dysfunctional sleep cognitions. Finally, a typical assessment protocol is outlined: sleep history, functional analysis, sleep diary monitoring, psychological screening, optional nocturnal polysomnography, and other discretionary procedures. This section sets the foundations for the cognitive-behavioral intervention described next.

The second section describes the treatment protocol—its format, duration, and content. This multifaceted intervention includes four therapy modules. The first two modules are behavior therapy, aimed at changing maladaptive sleep habits, and cognitive restructuring, designed to alter dysfunctional beliefs and attitudes about sleep. The third module provides sleep hygiene education; the fourth one reviews common medications prescribed for sleep, and provides a withdrawal plan for drug-dependent insomniacs. For each therapy component, a detailed description of the clinical procedures is provided, along with a rationale, methods of implementation, pitfalls to avoid, and problem-solving strategies to promote compliance.

The third section summarizes our knowledge about the clinical efficacy of this treatment program and of several other psychological therapies for the management of insomnia. Two treatment outcome data sets are reviewed. First, I discuss empirical findings from a clinical replication series of 100 insomnia sufferers treated in our clinic over the past few years. Also, the findings of a meta-analysis of 59 insomnia outcome studies conducted in various settings throughout the world are presented.

This book is a treatment manual for clinical practitioners. It builds upon psychological principles of behavior change. As such, it assumes basic knowledge and some training in psychotherapeutic interventions. It was written for psychologists, psychiatrists, social workers, nurses, trainees, and other health care practitioners. It is intended not only for sleep specialists, but for clinicians who wish to learn how to manage chronic insomnia effectively in their day-to-day practice.

Although a structured and multicomponent approach is advocated, this manual is not intended as a cookbook. Rather, the clinician is guided in integrating these procedures in a sequential fashion and in tailoring specific therapy components to individual patients' needs. Because insomnia is often associated with concomitant psychological and medical disorders, the clinician will find this time-limited treatment program helpful either as the sole intervention or as one therapy component integrated within a more global psychotherapeutic intervention geared toward other dysfunctions, such as anxiety, depression, or chronic pain. This manual provides a practical and structured approach with supporting didactic materials for both clinicians and patients.

CHARLES M. MORIN

# Contents

# I

# EVALUATION

# 1

# Insomnia: Scope of the Problem

This chapter presents an overview of insomnia and describes the scope of the problem. The nature of various insomnia complaints is examined, and the criteria used to evaluate their severity and clinical significance are outlined. The epidemiology of the disorder is reviewed, and its psychological, behavioral, and health correlates are summarized. Finally, clinical characteristics of insomnia sufferers seen in practice are highlighted.

## The Nature of Insomnia Complaints

"Insomnia" encompasses a wide variety of complaints typically reflecting unsatisfactory duration, efficiency, or quality of sleep. Presenting complaints often vary according to the moment of the night when sleep is most disturbed. They include problems with falling asleep at bedtime, waking up in the middle of the night, (and having difficulty in going back to sleep), and awakening too early in the morning. Clinicians and researchers refer to these conditions interchangeably as "sleep-onset" ("initial"), "sleep-maintenance" ("middle"), and "terminal" ("late") insomnia. These difficulties are not mutually exclusive, as a person may present with one, two, or all three problems. Sleep quality is usually described as light, restless, unrefreshing, or nonrestorative. Along with sleep complaints, reports of daytime sequelae (e.g., fatigue, tiredness, mood disturbances, social discomfort, and performance impairments) are extremely common. The complaint of insomnia is distinguished primarily from that of "hypersomnia," in which the predominant problem is staying awake during the day, and from "parasomnia," which implies abnormal behaviors during sleep.

## Definition and Severity Criteria

The clinical significance of insomnia is determined according to its severity, frequency, duration, and daytime sequelae. Sleep-onset insomnia requires

**3**

that the latency to sleep onset after turning the lights out be greater than 30 minutes. Sleep-maintenance insomnia involves either frequent and/or extended nocturnal awakenings totaling more than 30 minutes of wakefulness after sleep onset, or premature awakening in the morning with less than 6.5 hours of sleep. Mixed sleep-onset and sleep-maintenance insomnia involves a combination of difficulties with initiating and sustaining sleep. A sleep efficiency (time asleep divided by time spent in bed) of less than 85% is usually implied in making the diagnosis of insomnia. Although these criteria are useful to operationalize the various insomnias in outcome research (Lacks & Morin, 1992), two additional factors must be considered.

There are individual differences in the quantity of sleep needed to feel rested and function well during the day. About two-thirds of adults report between 7 and 8.5 hours of sleep per night (Gallup Organization, 1979; Kripke, Simons, Garfinkel, & Hammond, 1979). However, some people who are by nature "short sleepers" and get by with 4–5 hours of sleep per night may not suffer from insomnia, whereas others who are "long sleepers" and require 9–10 hours of sleep may still complain of insomnia. Accordingly, insomnia is not merely a reflection of diminished sleep, and total sleep time alone is not a good index of its severity. Measures of sleep-onset latency, wake after sleep onset, or sleep efficiency represent more clinically meaningful indices of difficulties in initiating or maintaining sleep.

Another important issue is that insomnia is a fairly subjective phenomenon that is not always corroborated by objective evidence (Borkovec, 1982). For instance, it is well established that poor sleepers tend to overestimate sleep-onset latency and wake after sleep onset, and to underestimate sleep duration, compared to polysomnography (Coates et al., 1982). These discrepancies are present in both good and poor sleepers, though they are significantly more pronounced in the latter group. In addition, some people complaining of insomnia fail to show any objective feature of abnormal sleep. There is a substantial overlap between these individuals (subjective insomniacs) and those whose complaint is corroborated by objective findings (psychophysiological insomniacs). For now, let us assume that the intensity of insomnia complaints is sometimes amplified and may not always reflect absolute levels of sleep disturbances measured by polysomnography.

Even so, sleep may still be perceived as qualitatively deficient. For example, some people describe their phenomenological experience of a poor night's sleep as that of being in a "twilight zone" (half awake, half asleep) all night long. There is no major problem with initiating or maintaining sleep, but its quality is described as light and nonrestorative, with persisting intrusive thoughts preventing the natural progression to a deep slumber. Such a complaint is sometimes associated with a condition called "alpha–delta" sleep, that is, frequent intrusion of alpha rhythms (wakefulness) into non-rapid-eye-movement sleep stages. It is more difficult to quantify unless it can be correlated with polysomnographic data and the amount of time spent in various sleep stages.

The frequency and duration of the sleep problem must be considered in the severity equation. Virtually everyone experiences an occasional poor night's sleep, and as such would not necessarily be considered insomniac. In general, insomnia experts agree that sleep difficulties must be experienced three or more nights per week to be clinically significant. The duration of the current problem is also important, as transient and persistent insomnia may have different etiological and treatment implications. Almost everyone encounters situational sleep disturbances as a result of such stressful life events as a death in the family, financial problems, change of job, or a strained marital relationship. Insomnia lasting less than 1 month is considered transient or situational in nature; generally, though not always, it resolves itself after the individual has adjusted to the stressful events. Insomnia lasting between 1 and 6 months is considered short-term or subacute, and when it persists for more than 6 months it is classified as chronic (*International Classification of Sleep Disorders* [ICSD]; American Sleep Disorders Association [ASDA], 1990). In clinical practice, the majority of insomnia sufferers seek specialized treatment only after they have endured such difficulties for several years (Morin, Stone, McDonald, & Jones, 1992).

The extent to which psychological, social, and occupational functioning are affected by chronic insomnia is one of the most important criteria in determining its clinical significance. Diminished sleep in the absence of any sequelae has different treatment implications than when it is accompanied by daytime impairments. According to the fourth edition of the *Diagnostic and Statistical Manual of Mental Disorders* (DSM-IV; American Psychiatric Association [APA], in press), the sleep disturbance must be associated with daytime fatigue or impaired functioning to make a diagnosis of insomnia. Further, the sleep disturbance (or daytime sequelae) must cause significant impairment in social or occupational functioning, or cause marked distress. Although objective evidence of daytime sequelae is often lacking, a patient's subjective perception of such deficits can cause psychological distress and perpetuate sleep difficulties.

Several studies have compared the sleep patterns of chronic insomniacs with those of normal controls (Coates et al., 1982; Gillin, Duncan, Pettigrew, Frankel, & Snyder, 1979; Hauri & Fisher, 1986; A. Kales et al., 1984). Depending on the subjects' age and the underlying problem (sleep-onset, sleep-maintenance, or mixed insomnia), insomniacs show longer sleep-onset latencies, more time awake after sleep onset, less total sleep, and a lower sleep efficiency than controls. These differences are obtained whether based on subjective reports (Espie, Monk, Hood, & Lindsay, 1988; Morin & Gramling, 1989) or on polysomnography, though in the latter case the magnitude of the between-group differences (poor vs. good sleepers) are smaller. On a more qualitative basis, insomniacs spend more time in stage 1 sleep, spend less time in stages 3–4 sleep, and display more frequent stage shifts through the night than do normal controls. Interestingly, difficulties in initiating and maintaining sleep seen in psychophysiological insomniacs are fairly similar to those observed in patients with anxiety or affective disorders (Hauri & Fisher, 1986; Reynolds, Shaw, Newton, Coble, & Kupfer, 1983; Reynolds et al., 1984; Rosa, Bonnet, & Kramer, 1983); perhaps this similarity suggests a common underlying thread to these conditions.

In summary, when the DSM-IV and ICSD criteria are combined with those typically used in clinical research, persistent insomnia is defined as follows:

1.  Subjective complaints of poor sleep.
2.  Difficulties in initiating and/or maintaining sleep, whereby sleep-onset latency and/or wake after sleep onset is greater than 30 minutes; sleep efficiency is lower than 85%.
3.  Sleep difficulties are present 3 or more nights per week.
4.  Duration of insomnia is longer than 6 months.
5.  Subjective report of at least one daytime sequela attributed to poor sleep: fatigue, performance impairment, or mood disturbances.
6.  The sleep disturbance (or daytime sequelae) causes significant impairment in social or occupational functioning, or causes marked distress.

## Epidemiology

Insomnia is a widespread problem affecting essentially everyone at one period or another in a lifetime. It is the most common of all sleep disorders (Bixler, Kales, Soldatos, Kales, & Healy, 1979) and perhaps the most frequent health complaint after pain. Epidemiological surveys conducted in North America and in Europe have yielded prevalence rates ranging from a conservative 2% (Liljenberg, Almqvist, Hetta, Roos, & Agren, 1989) to an overwhelming 42.5% (Bixler, Kales, Soldatos, et al., 1979). The extensive variability in these figures is attributable to the use of different definitions of insomnia and different data collection techniques (questionnaires vs. phone interviews vs. face-to-face interviews).

A recent Gallup survey based on 1,950 phone interviews found that 36% of Americans suffer from some type of sleep problem, with 27% of respondents reporting occasional insomnia and 9% saying that their sleep difficulty occurs on a regular, chronic basis (Gallup Organization, 1991). Data from two large community surveys based on home interviews have yielded similar prevalence rates. According to the National Survey of Psychotherapeutic Drug Use, about 35% of the adult population is afflicted by insomnia during the course of a year (Mellinger, Balter, & Uhlenhuth, 1985). Of these, half experience their sleep problem as serious, whereas the remaining perceive theirs as mild and transient. Using a more operational definition, the National Institute of Mental Health (NIMH) Epidemiologic Catchment Area study yielded a 10.2% prevalence rate of serious insomnia, in comparison to 3.2% for hypersomnia (Ford & Kamerow, 1989). Insomnia was defined as a problem in falling asleep or staying asleep for 2 weeks or more in the past 6 months that was not attributable to physical illnesses, medications, or substance abuse, and for which the respondents had told a professional about it, taken medication for it, or stated that it interfered significantly with their lives. Of the initial 10.2% with insomnia, 31% continued to report insomnia at a second interview conducted 1 year later, yielding a 3% rate of chronic insomnia. This figure is comparable to other studies using an even more stringent definition, such as problems with falling asleep or staying asleep almost every night, in which sleep-onset latency or wake after sleep onset exceeded 30 minutes (Bliwise, King, Harris, & Haskell, 1992; Liljenberg et al., 1989).

Surveys of physicians indicate that 19% of medical outpatients complain of insomnia (Bixler, Kales, & Soldatos, 1979). Although only 5% of patients specifically visit a health professional for sleep problem, 28% discuss sleep problems during visits for other purpose (Gallup Organization, 1991), and 40–60% acknowledge sleep problems when specifically asked about it (Dement, 1991a). Another survey found that of 100 consecutive medical inpatients referred for psychiatric consultation, 72 were diagnosed with insomnia of various origins (Berlin, Litovitz, Diaz, & Ahmed, 1984). In a case series of more than 5,000 patients evaluated at 11 sleep disorders centers across the United States, 31% were diagnosed with insomnia in comparison to 52% with hypersomnia, 15% with parasomnias, and 3% with sleep–wake schedule problems (Coleman et al., 1982). The higher prevalence of hypersomnia in that sample is somewhat misleading, since several of the participating centers specialized in the treatment of disorders such as sleep apnea and narcolepsy, whose primary symptom is excessive daytime sleepiness.

Sleep disturbances are by no means restricted to adults (Mindell, 1993). More than 30% of preschool children, 26% of pediatric patients, and 15% of adolescents suffer from sleep disruptions (Lozoff, Wolf, & Davis, 1985; Coates & Thoresen, 1981). Although children rarely complain of insomnia, their temper tantrums at bedtime or prolonged awakenings and crying in the middle of the night often cause parental distress (Ferber, 1985; Wolfson, Lacks, & Futterman, 1992). In school-age children, sleep disruptions may cause social, behavioral, and learning problems, and perhaps predispose the children to adulthood insomnia (Cashman & McCann, 1988). In adolescents, sleep disturbance is often accompanied by the same emotional correlates as those manifested in adults (Price, Coates, Thoresen, & Grinstead, 1978). Nightmares, night terrors, sleepwalking, and sleep talking are especially common among children (see Mindell, 1993), though most of these parasomnias are outgrown by late adolescence.

The complaint of insomnia is associated with several demographic variables, including age, gender, and occupational and socioeconomic status. The strongest relationship is with age. More than 25% of people age 65 or older report sleep disruptions (Mellinger et al., 1985). The nature of these complaints changes with aging. Sleep-onset difficulties are more frequent among younger adults, whereas sleep-maintenance problems, such as nocturnal and early-morning awakenings, are especially common in late life (Bixler, Kales, Soldatos, et al., 1979; Mellinger et al., 1985). Although older adults are not exempt from sleep-onset insomnia, their main problem is in sustaining sleep. Deteriorating health may partially account for the increased prevalence of sleep disturbances with aging, but even when medical factors are covaried out, insomnia remains a significant concern for many seniors (Bliwise et al., 1992; Morin & Gramling, 1989).

Insomnia complaints are twice as common in women as in men (Bixler, Kales, Soldatos, et al., 1979). The gender difference may indicate a greater willingness among women to acknowledge and seek treatment for insomnia, but it may also reflect a more accurate perception of disturbed sleep. For example, objective and subjective measures of sleep parameters are more strongly correlated in older women than in men (Hoch et al., 1987). Paradoxically, in noncomplaining older adults, men display more pathologies (sleep apnea, periodic limb movements) than women (Reynolds et al., 1985). Insomnia complaints are more common among homemakers, the unemployed, separated and widowed individuals, and people living alone (Bixler, Kales, Soldatos, et al., 1979; Ford & Kamerow, 1989). Their incidence is inversely related to educational and socioeconomic levels, though this finding has not been consistent across surveys (Gallup Organization, 1991). Disturbed sleep and psychopathology tend to covary, and the combination of poor education, unemployment, and poor psychological adjustment may all contribute to increase the vulnerability to insomnia. Nevertheless, it is by no means restricted to people of lower socioeconomic levels. Many wealthy and highly successful individuals also suffer from insomnia, though they may be less inclined to acknowledge it, for such a problem is perceived by some as a sign of weakness and lack of control.

## Use of Sleeping Aids

The widespread use of sleeping aids is a good index of the scope of insomnia problems. According to a recent Gallup survey commissioned by the National Sleep Foundation (Gallup Organization, 1991), 20% of those who complained of insomnia had received a prescription for a sleeping pill at some time in the past. In the NIMH survey of psychotherapeutic drug use, 7.1%, or 15% of those reporting serious insomnia, had used either a prescribed (4.3%) or over-the-counter (3.1%) sleeping aid within the previous year (Mellinger et al., 1985). Of those, 11% had used medications regularly for more than 1 year. Among the various prescribed sleep-promoting agents, 61% received hypnotics, 27% anxiolytics, and 11% antidepressants. Older people, particularly women, are more likely to use sleep-promoting drugs (Mellinger et al., 1985). In a study of seniors living at home, 16% were currently taking hypnotic drugs, and many of these had done so for more than a year (Morgan, Dallosso, Ebrahim, Arie, & Fentem, 1988). In nursing facilities in the 1970s, 94% of the elderly residents had been prescribed sedative–hypnotics at a given time (U.S. Public Health Service, 1976). Overall, 39% of prescriptions for hypnotics were written for persons over 60 years of age, even though this group represented only 12% of the population at that time (Institute of Medicine, 1979). Physicians' prescribing practices for sleep-related problems are more conservative nowadays, and the use of hypnotics has declined in the last 20 years. Nonetheless, many people self-medicate their sleep problems with alcohol and/or over-the-counter remedies. The use of sleeping aids strictly on a prophylactic basis is not uncommon. In one survey, more than one-third of those who reported they seldom had trouble sleeping nevertheless acknowledged that they often used sleeping pills (Kripke et al., 1979).

## The Impact of Chronic Insomnia

Sleep disturbances can adversely affect a person's life, causing significant psychosocial, occupational, and health repercussions. For example, chronic insomnia sufferers report more impaired concentration and memory, and more difficulty in accomplishing needed tasks during the day, than do good sleepers. They have more difficulty in coping with minor irritations and report less enjoyment of family and social relationships; they also feel less well physically. Finally, they are more than twice as likely (5% vs. 2%) as noninsomniacs to report motor vehicle accidents in which fatigue was a factor (Gallup Organization, 1991). Although these findings do not imply causality, insomnia is clearly not a benign problem. It has a detrimental effect on quality of life and psychological well-being. These and other correlates are reviewed below.

## Psychological Correlates

Individuals with sleep disturbances are more likely to display concomitant psychological distress than those without sleep complaints (Mellinger et al.,

1985). Although not everyone worries about disturbed sleep, especially when it is transient in nature, those who have to struggle nightly with this problem experience such mood disturbances as irritability, tension, helplessness, and a general sense of dysphoria. The unpredictable nature of sleep is often associated with performance anxiety, and the perception of losing control is linked with a sense of learned helplessness. The natural course of insomnia is often one that begins with anxiety resulting from stressful life events, then insomnia, and finally depression. For other people, however, the initial precipitating event may trigger depression and then insomnia. Nonetheless, longitudinal data suggest that individuals whose insomnia is left untreated for over 1 year are more likely to develop major depression than either normal controls or those whose insomnia has resolved during this time period (Ford & Kamerow, 1989).

Several investigations have examined the daytime concomitants of poor sleep. For example, the subjective effects of sleep quality were explored by comparing ratings of several dimensions of daytime functioning after both a poor and a good night's sleep (Zammit, 1988). Four factors describing the perceived sequelae of poor sleep were identified: dysphoria (feeling unhappy, low energy, social withdrawal, low interest, and inattentiveness); cognitive inefficiency (poor concentration, feeling tired, mental slowness, lethargy); motor impairment (accident proneness, feeling clumsy); and social discomfort (feeling easily intimidated by others, wanting to avoid others). Similar results were obtained by other researchers (J.D. Kales et al., 1984; Marchini, Coates, Magistad, & Waldum, 1983). Unfortunately, these findings are strictly based on cross-sectional studies, and because mood disturbances may precipitate nocturnal sleep difficulties, the only relationship that can be implied is covariation.

Several studies using the Minnesota Multiphasic Personality Inventory (MMPI) have been conducted to describe the personality profiles of insomniacs (Edinger, Stout, & Hoelscher, 1988; A. Kales, Caldwell, Soldatos, Bixler, & Kales, 1983; Shealy, Lowe, & Ritzler, 1980). Two clusters (2–7–3, 1–2–3) have been reported with some consistency across investigations. These profiles suggest depressed and anxious moods; a cognitive style characterized by excessive worrying and obsessive ruminations; internalization of psychological conflicts; and preoccupations with one's health. Elevation of scale 8, reflecting a sense of social alienation, has also been noted. Although MMPI data are valuable for understanding the psychological "make-up" of chronic insomniacs as a group, not all insomniacs display concurrent psychopathology. Furthermore, these data do not provide information about the direction of the relationship between psychological and sleep disturbances.

In conclusion, there is a strong relationship between sleep and emotional disturbances, though the extent to which one is the cause and which is the consequence is unclear. Nonetheless, the overall evidence indicates that insomnia causes psychological distress in some individuals, and that in those already afflicted by emotional problems, chronically disturbed sleep may only potentiate these difficulties.

## Behavioral Correlates

A frequent concern among insomniacs is the extent to which their behavioral or cognitive performance is impaired as a result of poor sleep. Although numerous studies have evaluated performance decrements following experimental sleep deprivation (see Johnson, 1982), very few have been conducted with chronic insomniacs. In otherwise normal sleepers, prolonged sleep loss is generally followed by impaired performance on measures of cognitive and psychomotor skills requiring sustained attention (e.g. four-choice reaction time, digit–symbol substitution, auditory vigilance, logical reasoning, arithmetic). However, findings on the aftereffects of a poor night's sleep in insomniacs are inconsistent. One study of neuropsychological functioning in older insomniacs revealed no impairment of cognitive and psychomotor performance (Stone, Morin, Hart, Remsberg, & Mercer, 1992). Other studies also found no difference between poor and good sleepers on baseline measures of reaction time and motor speed prior to drug treatments (Church & Johnson, 1979; Seidel et al., 1984), whereas still others reported impaired vigilance, concentration, and lower achievement scores in poor sleepers (Spinweber & Johnson, 1982; Sugerman, Stern, & Walsh, 1985; Webb & Levy, 1982).

Collectively, these results suggest that chronic sleep disturbances may impair waking functions but that the deficits are subtle and inconsistent across individuals. Caution is advised before generalizing from these time-limited laboratory experiments to real-life situations, however, as several variables may mediate performance under these different circumstances. First, the duration and timing of testing is critical. Psychomotor and cognitive deficits become more noticeable toward the end of prolonged and nonstimulating tasks. Performance is more impaired in the morning than in the afternoon or evening (Schneider-Helmert, 1987), perhaps owing to more disturbed mood at this time of the day. Furthermore, a subject's motivation and the demand characteristics of an experimental situation may override deficits that would otherwise become apparent in real-life situations. Finally, although there may be discrepancies between perceived and objective deficits, we have yet to develop measures that are sensitive enough to detect subtle performance decrements. The use of unobtrusive measures in naturalistic situations that tap targets more sensitive to sleep loss (e.g., motivation, initiative, creativity) might yield more meaningful data.

Reports of fatigue, tiredness, or drowsiness almost always accompany insomnia complaints. Sleepiness is the most predictable consequence of sleep deprivation. In chronic insomniacs, however, the impact of disturbed sleep on daytime alertness is equivocal. Several studies have used the Multiple Sleep Latency Test (MSLT) to examine this issue. Individuals are offered five 20-minute naps at 2-hour intervals throughout the day, and the speed with which they fall asleep provides an objective measure of sleepiness. Despite more disturbed sleep, insomniacs are no more sleepy (Seidel et al., 1984) and perhaps even more alert during the day (Stepanski, Zorick, Roehrs, Young, & Roth, 1988) than control subjects. The chronic hyperarousal state that characterizes psychophysiological insomniacs throughout the 24-hour cycle may explain these paradoxical findings. Excessive arousal impedes the ability to fall asleep not only at night but also during the day. As such, insomniacs typically fall asleep more easily in nonsleeping environments and when they are not attempting to do so. Excessive motivation to fall asleep delays its onset (Shaffer, Dickel, Marik, & Slak, 1985), and the instructional demand of the MSLT (i.e., "Try to go to sleep") may simply induce performance anxiety. Thus, the MSLT data for insomniacs may reflect an underlying state of hyperarousal surrounding the presleep period and the sleep environment, rather than being truly indicative of alertness.

A more puzzling finding is that subjective insomniacs—that is, those without objective evidence of disturbed sleep—are more sleepy during the day than either objective insomniacs or good sleepers (Sugerman et al., 1985). Although this phenomenon is difficult to explain, it is plausible that this subgroup appraises sleep quality and duration in a retrospective fashion. After experiencing daytime sleepiness or performance impairments, these individuals may misattribute such deficits to poor sleep, whereas other factors might well have caused these.

Unlike the MSLT, pupillometric assessment indicates that insomniacs are less alert than normal controls (Lichstein, Johnson, Gupta, O'Laughlin, & Dykstra, 1992). This assessment procedure, which involves measurements of pupil size and stability in the dark, has been shown to detect improved alertness following behavioral treatment of insomnia (Nicassio & Bootzin, 1974). However, not unlike the discrepancies between subjective and objective measures of nocturnal sleep, insomniacs' ratings of daytime sleepiness are not corroborated by either MSLT or pupillometric assessment (Lichstein et al., 1992; Seidel et al., 1984). Thus, instead of being truly sleepy by day, insomniacs may be mislabeling their internal state; this might be more accurately described as fatigue or tiredness than as true sleepiness.

## Health Correlates

Insomnia sufferers seen in clinical practice often express concerns about the detrimental impact of poor sleep on their health, and quite frequently attribute somatic problems to lack of sleep. Evidence from epidemiological, cross-sectional, and longitudinal studies suggests a strong association between sleep and other somatic complaints, though there is no clear cause-and-effect relationship. For example, insomniacs report more health problems, more frequent hospitalizations, and more limitations of their work capacity because of sleep problems than good sleepers serving as controls (Bixler, Kales, Soldatos, et al., 1979; J.D. Kales et al., 1984). Mellinger et al. (1985) found that 53% of those with serious insomnia reported two or more health problems during the 12 months preceding the survey, in comparison to a base rate of 32% for the entire sample. In a survey of Swedish men, sleep complaints were twice as prevalent among those regularly attending medical examinations as among others (Gislason & Almqvist, 1987). Of 70 patients with a recent myocardial infarction, 39% reported having had insomnia for 2 weeks or longer prior to their infarction, suggesting that insomnia may be an early precursor of heart attacks in some individuals (Carney, Freedland, & Jaffe, 1990). In a longitudinal study, poor health status in elderly subjects was linked with more severe sleep disturbances, particularly early-morning awakenings (Rodin, McAvay, & Timko, 1988).

Physical complaints reported by insomniacs often have a psychosomatic connotation: tension headaches, gastrointestinal problems, nonspecific aches and pains, and allergies (J.D. Kales et al., 1984). This is not surprising, since insomnia itself is hypothesized to result from somatized tension and anxiety that are released into physiological channels. Whether or not insomnia sufferers have more physical illnesses, they are more preoccupied with their health and more likely to use health-related services than good sleepers (Ford & Kamerow, 1989; J.D. Kales et al., 1984; Morgan et al., 1988). It is unclear whether these preoccupations are justified or simply reflect underlying hypochondriacal tendancies.

Sleep duration is linked to longevity. In a large prospective survey of health-related habits, the American Cancer Society collected data from over 1 million Americans over a period of several years (Hammond, 1964). Data on sleep complaints, sleep durations, and use of sleeping pills were correlated with mortality rates obtained 6 years later (Kripke et al., 1979). Insomnia in itself was unrelated to mortality rate. However, subjects reporting either short (4 hours or less) or long (more than 10 hours) sleep durations had a mortality rate 1.5 to 2.0 times higher than those with a sleep duration falling in the 7- to 8-hour range. People using sleeping pills "often" also had a mortality rate 1.5 times higher than those who "never" used sleeping pills. These results should be interpreted cautiously because people who have excessively short or long sleep, or who use sleeping pills, often suffer from medical conditions (e.g., heart disease, diabetes, sleep apnea) that in themselves are associated with reduced longevity.

Sleep difficulties and disruptive nighttime behaviors are two of the most common reasons given by caregivers for placing elderly relatives in chronic care facilities (Sanford, 1975). The "sundown syndrome" in patients with Alzheimer's disease is characterized by nocturnal confusion, disorientation, and wandering despite fairly good functioning by day (Evans, 1987). This can produce great concern and disturbed sleep in family members who are attempting to manage these nocturnal behavioral problems. Among community-dwelling elderly males, insomnia is the strongest predictor of nursing home placement and exceeds that associated with cognitive impairment (Pollak, Perlick, Linsner, Wenston, & Hsieh, 1990).

In summary, insomnia is a widespread complaint affecting about 10% of the population on a chronic basis. It is more prevalent in women and in older people. It can adversely affect both physical and mental health. Although there is limited evidence to suggest a direct causal relationship among these factors, insomnia sufferers are more preoccupied with their health and report more recurrent somatic problems than do good sleepers. Chronic insomnia may induce emotional distress and increase the use of psychotropic medications and the risk of substance abuse. Economic repercussions are also evident in terms of diminished productivity, absenteeism from work, and the costs associated with greater utilization of health-related services. Whether or not the subjective complaints about insomnia and its daytime sequelae are amplified or objectively verifiable, chronic insomnia is a genuine clinical problem that diminishes the quality of life and causes considerable distress.

## Characteristics of Insomniacs Seeking Treatment

Insomnia may begin at any period of life, but the average age of onset clusters in the mid-30s for sleep-onset difficulties and the mid-50s for sleep-maintenance problems. It may be several years, however, before an individual seeks professional help. Most people with sleep problems have tried a host of self-remedies, such as a hot bath, a self-hypnosis tape, alcohol, or a variety of over-the-counter medications. When all of these have failed, they may have brought the problem to the attention of a primary care physician. Unfortunately, sleep complaints are often overlooked, ignored, or simply interpreted as symptoms of anxiety or depression. Until insomnia becomes a recurrent complaint, general medical practitioners may pay little attention to it. Dement (1991a) explains this paradox by saying that "doctors do not want to ask about sleep problems because they do not know what to do to alleviate them" (p. vii). When treatment is indeed initiated, prescription of a hypnotic is often the only recommendation. Of those consulting a physician specifically for insomnia, about one-half are prescribed sleeping pills (Bixler, Kales, & Soldatos, 1979).

Most patients seen in our clinic at the Medical College of Virginia are either self- or physician-referred individuals with mixed sleep-onset and sleep-maintenance insomnia, and about half of them are using some form of sleep aid. Their average insomnia duration is 12 years (Morin, Stone, et al., 1992). This chronicity is typical for either self- or physician-referred patients, as well as for community-recruited subjects who volunteer for treatment studies (Espie, 1991; J.D. Kales et al., 1984; Lacks & Powlishta, 1989; Stepanski et al., 1989). Although insomnia severity does not differ between patients who seek or do not seek treatment, those seen in therapy display a higher level of psychological distress (Stepanski et al., 1989). They express a great deal of dissatisfaction with their sleep and present in treatment with some features of anxiety and depression. Although they may not necessarily meet criteria for a diagnosable psychopathology, they express significant concerns about their sleep, and even more concerns about the impact of sleep loss on physical and mental health as well as on daytime functioning. Additional clinical features of insomniacs seen in treatment are discussed in later chapters.

# 2

## Basic Facts about Sleep

This chapter presents some basic facts about the nature of sleep and its measurement. Sleep stages and their cyclic pattern through the night are described. Normative developmental changes in sleep patterns are outlined and distinguished from pathological sleeplessness. The effects of prior sleep history, circadian rhythms, and drugs are summarized. The chapter concludes with a brief overview of the role and functions of sleep and the consequences of sleep loss. This review is not intended to be exhaustive; rather, it provides an introduction to the fundamentals of human sleep that should help the clinician place insomnia in its proper perspective. Because this book focuses on the psychological management of insomnia, the main emphasis is on the phenomenological, behavioral, and physiological substrates of sleep. Its neuroanatomical and neurochemical bases are not covered, as these have been well described elsewhere (Gaillard, 1985; Jones, 1989; Parkes, 1985).

### The Nature of Sleep

Researchers have identified two types of sleep: rapid-eye-movement (REM) and non-rapid-eye-movement (NREM) sleep. NREM sleep is further subdivided into four stages from stage 1, a very light sleep, to stage 4, the deepest stage of sleep. NREM sleep is also called "quiet" sleep, because most physiological functions are slowed down during this period of slumber (Hauri, 1982). Cognitive activity is minimal, but periodic body movements precede shifts from one sleep stage to another. For this reason, NREM sleep has been described as an "idling brain in a moveable body" (Carskadon & Dement, 1989). Conversely, REM sleep, also called "paradoxical," "active," or "fast" sleep, is characterized by electroencephalographic (EEG) activation, muscle atonia, and (as the name suggests) rapid eye movements. Vivid hallucinatory experiences (i.e., dreams) occur during REM sleep. Dreams may occasionally be recalled from NREM stages as well, but they lack the vivid visual imagery component and are more like daydreaming. Except for periodic muscle twitches, the body is essentially paralyzed during REM, which has been described as a "hyperactive brain in a paralyzed body" (Carskadon & Dement, 1989).

## Distribution of Sleep Stages through the Night

Sleep is not a random phenomenon. As illustrated in Figure 2.1, it is a highly structured and well-organized activity following a cyclic pattern. A normal young adult first enters sleep through NREM stages. From an initial state of drowsiness preceding sleep onset, the individual first drops to stage 1 and progressively moves into stage 2, stage 3, and stage 4. Stage 1 is a brief transitional phase bridging the gap between wakefulness and sleep and lasting only about 5 minutes. It is a very light sleep, and arousal threshold is correspondingly low. Stage 2 sleep, which lasts between 10 and 20 minutes during the initial cycle, is considered true or nonequivocal physiological sleep because it corresponds most closely to the phenomenological experience of sleep onset (Hauri & Olmstead, 1983). Stages 3 and 4, also called "delta" or "slow-wave" sleep, are the deepest stages of sleep. Consequently, arousal threshold is highest during this phase, which may last between 20 and 40 minutes in the first sleep cycle. This initial sequence is followed by a return from stage 4 to stage 3 and stage 2, leading to the first REM episode. The first REM period takes place 70–90 minutes after sleep onset and is usually of brief duration (5–15 minutes). On the average, four to five REM episodes of increasing duration occur throughout the night.

The duration of NREM–REM cycles is approximately 90 minutes, but may vary between 70 and 120 minutes. Delta or slow-wave sleep is predomi-

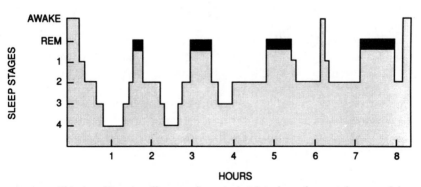

HOURS

**FIGURE 2.1.** This sleep histogram illustrates the typical night's sleep of a normal young adult.

nant in the first third of the night, whereas the proportion of REM sleep is much greater in the last third of the night. Whether bedtime is 9:00 P.M., 11:00 P.M., or 1:00 A.M., a typical night's sleep begins by a period of deep sleep followed by a period of REM sleep. When bedtime is pushed very late in the early morning hours, REM sleep may come quicker than usual, and delta sleep may consequently be delayed and shortened. In young adulthood, approximately 75% of the sleep time is spent in NREM and 25% in REM stages. Stage 1 makes up only about 5% of the sleep time, whereas about 50% is spent in stage 2 and 20% in deep sleep (stages 3–4). Although these figures are fairly precise for a healthy young adult, several factors (to be reviewed later) alter the proportion of time spent in each stage, as well as their distribution into the night.

Several phenomenological, behavioral, and physiological changes accompany the transition from wakefulness to sleep and the passage from NREM to REM sleep. The subjective experience of falling asleep is often different in good and poor sleepers. For example, cognitive activity may persist in insomniacs even after sleep onset. Consequently, insomniacs report more frequently than good sleepers being awake when their EEG tracings indicate stage 1 or even stage 2 sleep (Borkovec, Lane, & Van Oot, 1981; Coates et al., 1983). Amnesia for what happened just before falling asleep (Guilleminault & Dement, 1977) or upon waking up at night (Bonnet, 1983) is common. This phenomenon may explain why it is difficult to recall the exact moment of sleep onset or to remember phone calls in the middle of the night.

Behavioral responsivity to the environment gradually declines as sleep becomes more imminent. Because sleep onset is a gradual rather than a dichotomous process, some level of reactivity may persist even in stages 1 and 2 sleep (Ogilvie & Wilkinson, 1984; Ogilvie, Wilkinson, & Allison, 1989). Responsiveness to the environment is also influenced by the meaningfulness of the stimuli. People living around airports may learn to selectively block out noise from aircrafts while remaining responsive to a crying baby at night, suggesting that stimulus discrimination principles continue to operate even while asleep.

Physiological functions such as heart rate and respiratory rate slow down from wakefulness to NREM sleep. Blood pressure and oxygen consumption are also diminished. During REM sleep, however, pulse rate and respiratory rate rise (often above baseline levels) and become more irregular (Orem & Barnes, 1980). Transient blood pressure increases are frequently associated with phasic REM events. In males with normal erectile function, penile tumescence occurs with each REM episode (Ware, 1987), and in females blood flow to the vagina is increased. Thermoregulation is absent during REM sleep; that is, there is no shivering or sweating. Except for periodic muscle twitches, the body musculature is essentially paralyzed during REM. The diaphragm is also spared to preserve respiration.

## The Measurement of Sleep

The EEG, the electro-oculogram (EOG), and the electromyogram (EMG) are used to measure sleep. Surface electrodes attached to the scalp (EEG) and the skin (EOG, EMG) provide physiological signals that are amplified and simultaneously recorded on a polygraph. The EEG records brain wave activity from the central and occipital areas. The EOG measures a difference of electrical potential between the cornea and the retina; this difference is generated with each eye movement. The EMG monitors muscle tone, and its main recording site is the chin. The mastoid area can be used as well for evaluation of bruxism or temporomandibular joint dysfunctions (Carskadon & Rechtschaffen, 1989). Although these three variables are sufficient for monitoring and scoring sleep, a more extensive montage is often needed for diagnostic purposes.

Polysomnography involves several more channels that are used in the evaluation of breathing disorders or abnormal limb movements during sleep. Monitoring of nasal/oral airflow, respiratory effort, and oxygen saturation is used in the assessment and diagnosis of sleep apnea. The electrocardiogram (EKG) documents arrhythmias accompanying respiratory disturbances. EMG monitoring of the anterior tibialis muscles is used for detection of periodic leg movements during sleep. These electric potentials are also amplified and recorded on a polygraph. The standard monitoring speed is 10 millimeters per second, generating 1,200–1,500 feet of paper for an 8-hour study. Each page typically represents a 30-second epoch and is visually scored by a technician according to standard criteria for sleep (Rechtschaffen & Kales, 1968), respiration, leg movements, and any other abnormalities. A histogram similar to Figure 2.1 reproduces the entire night's sleep. Computer programs allow for the integration of these data in a summary report (e.g., sleep-onset latency, wake after sleep onset, sleep efficiency, percentage of sleep in each NREM stage, percentage of REM sleep, etc.). Automated-scoring programs are also available, though their concurrent validity with human scoring is still fairly poor.

NREM sleep is defined primarily by EEG criteria—that is, the frequency and the amplitude of brain waves (see Figure 2.2). Stage 1 is a transitional phase between wakefulness and sleep, and the EEG is characterized by brain waves of a low voltage and mixed frequency. These theta waves fall in the frequency band of 3–7 cycles per second, and gradually replace the alpha rhythm (8–12 cycles per second) typical of a relaxed wakeful state preceding sleep onset. Slow rolling-eye movements are usually present, and there is a slight decrease in EMG activity during the transition from drowsiness to sleep onset. Sleep onset is often accompanied by a hypnic jerk, a normal phenomenon involving a muscle contraction sometimes associated with an impression of falling down a cliff. During stage 2 sleep (see Figure 2.3), the EEG features K-complexes and sleep spindles (bursts of 12–14 cycles per second).

**Awake** – low voltage – random, fast

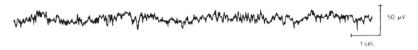

50 μV

1 sec.

**Drowsy** – 8 to 12 cps – alpha waves

**Stage 1** – 3 to 7 cps – theta waves

Theta Waves

**Stage 2** – 12 to 14 cps – sleep spindles and K complexes

Sleep Spindle

K Complex —

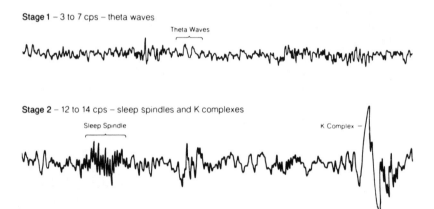

**Delta Sleep** – ½ to 2 cps – delta waves >75 μV

**REM Sleep** – low voltage – random, fast with sawtooth waves

Sawtooth Waves     Sawtooth Waves

**FIGURE 2.2.** EEG of sleep stages. From Hauri, P. J. (1982). *The sleep disorders.* Kalamazoo, MI: Upjohn. Copyright 1977 by The Upjohn Company. Reprinted by permission of the publisher and author.

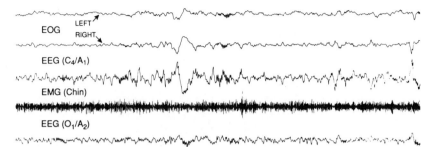

**FIGURE 2.3.** Polygraphic recording of stage 2 sleep. EOG, electro-oculogram (left eye and right eye); EMG, electromyogram (chin); EEG, electroencephalogram (central and occipital locations).

The EEG of stages 3 and 4, delta rhythm, is characterized by slow waves (0.5 to 2 cycles per second) with a high amplitude (i.e., >75 microvolts). Stage 3 is scored when a given 30-second epoch contains between 20% and 50% of delta waves, whereas stage 4 requires that more than 50% of an epoch meet these criteria. Slow-wave sleep (stages 3 and 4) is the deepest sleep, and arousal threshold is highest.

All three electrophysiological measures (EEG, EOG, and EMG) are needed to score REM sleep, which, as noted above, is characterized by EEG activation, muscle atonia, and rapid eye movements. Sawtooth brain wave patterns are interspersed in a background of EEG activation similar to that observed during wakefulness; this reflects the high level of mental activity unfolding during this sleep stage. Paradoxically, voluntary muscles are totally paralyzed during REM sleep. REM sleep is also subdivided into tonic and phasic components. The tonic background consists primarily of muscle atonia, whereas phasic events consist of periodic bursts of rapid eye movements, muscle twitches, and EEG sawtooth waves that occur throughout this stage. Arousal threshold is very variable in REM sleep.

## Developmental Changes across the Lifespan

Several developmental changes in sleep patterns occur over the course of the lifespan (see Figure 2.4). The proportion of time spent awake and asleep, and the amount of time spent in various stages, change across age groups (Roffward, Muzio, & Dement, 1966; Williams, Karacan, & Hursch, 1974; Webb, 1989). Total sleep time is highest in infancy and gradually declines, leveling off in young adulthood. Average sleep time per 24-hour cycle decreases from about 16–18 hours during infancy to 10–11 hours in early childhood and about 7–9 hours in the mid-20s. Nocturnal sleep is diminished in late life. However, daytime napping is common practice in older people, and when

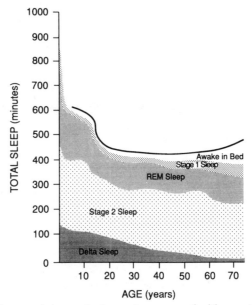

**FIGURE 2.4.** Developmental changes in sleep patterns across the lifespan. From Hauri, P. J. (1982). *The sleep disorders*. Kalamazoo, MI: Upjohn. Copyright 1977 by The Upjohn Company. Reprinted by permission of the publisher and author.

diurnal sleep is added to nighttime sleep, the amount of sleep per 24-hour period remains fairly stable from middle age to late life. Older people spend more time awake in bed. Consequently, sleep efficiency, or the ratio of time asleep to the total time spent in bed, is significantly decreased in late life. Contrary to the commonly held belief that sleep needs decrease with aging, the ability to sustain sleep uninterruptedly through the night, rather than sleep needs per se, may be what diminishes. This process is analogous to natural age-related declines of some physical and cognitive skills. The sleep pattern of the "very old" is characterized by polyphasic sleep–wake cycles. Instead of being consolidated in one period, their sleep (6–8 hours total) is obtained in two to four episodes; this pattern is developmentally similar to the polyphasic sleep cycle of infants (Dement, Miles, & Carskadon, 1982).

The proportion of time spent in NREM and REM sleep stages is age-dependent. The most significant of these changes, reflecting maturational processes, occur from infancy to late adolescence. Newborn babies spend about 50% of their sleep time in REM sleep. Infants go immediately into REM sleep, whereas adults enter sleep first through NREM. The percentage of REM sleep is stabilized by late adolescence (about 20–25%) and remains essentially unchanged until late life, when a slight decrease is noted. REM latency is also shorter and REM sleep is more evenly distributed throughout the night in older than in younger people (Reynolds et al., 1985). From puberty on, the proportion of stage 2 sleep remains fairly consistent across age groups. As people grow older, there is an increase in stage 1 sleep and a corresponding decrease in stages 3 and 4. Diminished slow-wave sleep is very gradual and fairly consistent from childhood to an older age.

These changes are accompanied by more frequent and longer nocturnal awakenings in older people (Webb & Campbell, 1980). Subjectively, these changes are experienced as lighter and more fragmented sleep, which may account for the increased prevalence of insomnia complaints in late life. Increases in physical illnesses (pain), medication use, and other sleep pathologies (sleep apnea, myoclonus) with aging (Ancoli-Israel, Kripke, Mason, & Messin, 1981; Gislason & Almqvist, 1987; Regenstein, 1980) exacerbate these complaints in older adults. Nevertheless, age, alone or in combination with health problems, cannot account for all insomnia problems in seniors (Morin & Gramling, 1989). Behavioral and cognitive factors are also involved in late-life insomnia, perhaps even to a greater extent than in insomnia at earlier ages.

## Factors Altering the Sleep Architecture

In addition to age or maturation, which is the most important factor modifying the sleep structure, sleep is affected by other variables: individual differences, prior sleep history, circadian rhythms, drugs, lifestyles, and psychopathology. The influence of some of these factors on the propensity to fall asleep, the duration of sleep, the proportion of time spent in each stage, and stage distribution throughout the night are now briefly reviewed.

### Sleep History

The duration and quality of sleep are dependent upon prior sleep history. Sleep deprivation experiments have shown that after sleep loss, several parameters are altered during the subsequent recovery period. The latency to sleep onset is inversely proportional to the length of the prior wake episode; that is, the longer one has been awake, the faster sleep onset occurs (Webb & Agnew, 1974). Sleep duration and percentage of slow-wave sleep are increased following sleep deprivation (Webb & Agnew, 1971). There is not, however, a linear relationship between the amount of sleep loss and the subsequent sleep length. If a person who usually gets 7 hours of sleep per night is kept awake for two nights, there will not be a need for 21 hours of sleep on the following night. Approximately one-third of the total sleep loss is usually recovered when a subject has the opportunity to sleep as long as desired.

Clinically, this is an important point to keep in mind when working with insomniacs, since these individuals often hold strong beliefs for the absolute need to make up on weekends for sleep loss suffered on weekdays. Laboratory experiments have shown that selective deprivation of a particular sleep stage leads to an increase in that stage on recovery nights. This "rebound phenomenon" is best illustrated with patients using antidepressant medications, which are known to suppress REM sleep. Abrupt drug discontinuation leads to an increased proportion, often exceeding baseline level, of that particular sleep stage. In patients with sleep apnea, there is often a chronic sleep fragmentation decreasing both REM and slow-wave sleep. The first few nights after the breathing disorder is corrected, exceedingly high proportions of these two stages are noted. After total sleep deprivation, slow-wave sleep is usually recovered first, followed by REM sleep.

## Circadian Factors

Chronobiological research has identified several biological and behavioral functions that are governed according to circadian (meaning "about a day") principles. The basic rest–activity cycle is a prime example of rhythmic behavior occuring on approximately a 24-hour interval. It is regulated by the interplay of internal biological "clocks" and environmental time markers. The suprachiasmatic nuclei, subcortical structures located in the hypothalamus, serve as an endogenous circadian oscillator. This clock is like a pendulum that is synchronized by several environmental time cues ("zeitgebers"). In humans, these time cues include social contacts, mealtimes, work schedules, and (most importantly) the light–dark cycle (Parkes, 1985). The sleep–wake cycle follows a circadian periodicity, which is dependent upon both intrinsic and extrinsic influences. In turn, these factors also determine the propensity to fall asleep, the duration of sleep, and the likelihood of entering particular sleep stages.

Temporal isolation studies have shown that young adults have a natural tendency to function not on a 24-hour but on a 25-hour day. These experiments are carried out in specially designed apartments without any cues as to the time of day (Weitzman, Czeisler, Zimmerman, Ronda, & Knauer, 1982; Wever, 1979). Clocks are removed, and ambient illumination is controlled by the subjects. The subjects are free to select the time they eat, go to bed, and arise. Under these "free-running" conditions, young adults tend to choose a sleep–wake cycle that is lengthened to about 25 hours (Czeisler, Weitzman, Moore-Ede, Zimmerman, & Knauer, 1980). This periodicity, however, fluctuates from person to person, and is considerably shorter than 24 hours in older people. Nevertheless, the natural tendency to function on a day slightly longer than 24 hours may explain why it is easier to rotate from a day to an evening shift than to a night shift, or easier to travel westbound than eastbound. It is simply easier to lengthen our days by fighting sleepiness than to shorten them by forcing sleep. Under normal or "entrained" conditions, humans constantly reset their internal clock by using environmental cues, so that the sleep–wake cycle operates in harmony with the night–day cycle.

Of the various biological functions (e.g., body temperature; secretion of growth hormone, cortisol, and melatonin) controlled by circadian rhythm principles, core body temperature is the one most relevant to understanding insomnia. It has a very stable rhythm and is strongly linked to the periodicity of sleep and wakefulness (see Figure 2.5). Body temperature is lowest in the early-morning hours, starts rising before awakening, peaks in early evening, and begins declining at about 11:00 P.M. This rhythm is closely tied to alertness–sleepiness (Monk, Leng, Folkard, & Weitzman, 1983). Alertness is maximum on the rising slope of the temperature curve, and sleepiness is greatest at its trough. A slight temperature decline in midafternoon is associated with a second prime time for falling asleep, suggesting that the postlunch dip is related to temperature change rather than to a full stomach (Richardson, Carskadon, Orav, & Dement, 1982). In prolonged isolation experiments, the temperature cycle (about 25 hours) splits off from the sleep–wake cycle, which is considerably longer, as discussed above.

Recent research has linked some insomnia subtypes to abnormal circadian rhythm of body temperature. For example, certain types of sleep-onset insomnia may arise from a delay in the temperature rhythm (Morris, Lack, & Dawson, 1990). Insomniacs also display higher temperature than good sleepers and less variation in their temperature curve throughout the 24-hour period. Under free-running conditions (i.e., no time cues, no time constraints), bedtime decisions are closely linked with a decline in temperature, and decisions about wake time occur shortly after temperature begins to rise

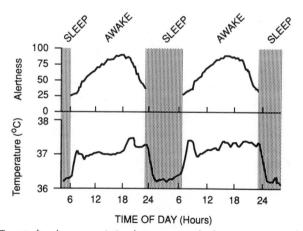

**FIGURE 2.5.** Twenty-four-hour covariation between core body temperature and alertness–sleepiness. From Coleman, R. M. (1986). *Wide awake at 3:00 a.m.: By choice or by chance?* New York: Freeman & Co. Copyright 1986 by Richard M. Coleman. Reprinted by permission of the author.

(Monk & Moline, 1989). Violations of these circadian principles alter the sleep episode by shortening its length and impairing its continuity.

The clock time determines not only the speed of sleep onset but also the likelihood of entering certain sleep stages. The propensity for REM sleep is highest in the early-morning hours, regardless of the duration of the prior wake episode, whereas slow-wave sleep is more dependent on the wake episode's duration. Accordingly, the timing of a daytime nap influences the type of sleep obtained. REM sleep is more likely to occur during a morning nap, because it is more like a continuation of the previous night's sleep. Conversely, an afternoon or evening nap, which is similar to the beginning of a normal night's sleep, is more likely to be made up of slow-wave sleep. There is a corresponding decrease of that stage in the subsequent night.

Chronobiological research has enhanced our understanding of etiological mechanisms involved in sleep–wake schedule disorders. Several types of insomnia are caused by a desynchronization between one's biological clock and the desired sleep–wake schedule, often resulting in sleeplessness at night and sleepiness during the day. The most common include insomnia as a result of work shift changes; jet lag following transmeridian flights; and phase-delay or phase-advance syndromes. These disorders are discussed in the next chapter.

## Drugs

Several drugs cause insomnia, others cause hypersomnia, and yet others selectively suppress some sleep stages. Table 2.1 summarizes the effects of several drugs on selected sleep parameters (A. Kales & Kales, 1984; Nicholson, Bradley, & Pascoe, 1989). These effects vary according to the schedule of administration, with those drugs consumed close to bedtime having the greatest impact on sleep. The effects observed under acute administration may also change with chronic use.

Sleep-promoting medications, particularly the benzodiazepines, increase stages 1 and 2 sleep and decrease slow-wave sleep. Their effects on REM sleep are variable and depend upon the specific pharmacological agent used. Long-acting agents may cause residual daytime sleepiness, whereas withdrawal from short-acting benzodiazepines typically causes insomnia (Gillin, Spinweber, & Johnson, 1989; A. Kales & Kales, 1984). Antidepressant drugs, including tricyclics, monoamine oxidase inhibitors, and the so-called "second-generation" drugs, have powerful REM-suppressing effects. Although some tricyclics (amitriptyline, doxepin) have sedating properties and may hasten sleep induction when given at bedtime, others (imipramine, protriptyline) are more energizing and delay its onset. Fluoxetine (Prozac) is well known to cause insomnia. Neuroleptics may initially increase stages 3–4 sleep and decrease wake after sleep onset, but these effects disappear with chronic use. Lithium has similar short-term effects: It increases slow-wave sleep and decreases wake after sleep onset and REM sleep. The long-term effects of most of these psychotropic medications is unknown.

Several drugs prescribed for medical disorders may secondarily alter sleep (A. Kales & Kales, 1984; Mitler, Poceta, Menn, & Erman, 1991). Most steroids (e.g., prednisone) used to control inflammation produce insomnia. Some bronchodilators (e.g., theophylline) prescribed in the treatment of asthma have a stimulating effect and often lead to sleep difficulties when used at bedtime. Although antihypertensive medications usually cause daytime sedation, some of the beta-blockers (propranolol, methyldopa, clonidine) increase sleep-onset latency and wake after sleep onset (Rosen & Kostis, 1985; Betts & Alford, 1983). Another paradoxical finding is that these drugs generally decrease the amount of REM sleep but that patients often complain of nightmares. Though commonly used for their sedating side effects, most antihistamines only cause daytime drowsiness; they have limited potential as sleep aids (Roehrs, Tietz, Zorick, & Roth, 1984).

Almost any central nervous system stimulant interferes with the initiation and maintenance of sleep. Caffeine and nicotine are both central nervous system stimulants, and they fragment sleep; appetite-suppressant medications have similar effects. Amphetamines and cocaine impair both sleep onset and maintenance, and selectively suppress REM sleep. Alcohol, a central nervous system depressant, may initially deepen sleep and decrease the percentage of REM sleep early in the night, but it is usually followed in the latter part of the night by REM rebound, impairment of sleep continuity,

**TABLE 2.1.** The Effects of Drugs on Selected Sleep Parameters

| Drugs | SOL | WASO | TST | REM | SWS | EDS |
|-------|-----|------|-----|-----|-----|-----|
| Benzodiazepines | ↓ | ↓ | ↑ | ? | ↓ | ↑ |
| Antidepressants | ? | ? | ? | ↓ | ? | ? |
| Neuroleptics | ↓ | ↓ | ? | ↓ | ↑ | ↑ |
| Lithium | ? | ↓ | ? | ↓ | ↑ | ? |
| Beta-blockers | ↑ | ↑ | ? | ↓ | ? | ↑ |
| Steroids | ↑ | ↑ | ↓ | ? | ? | ↓ |
| Bronchodilators | ↑ | ↑ | ↓ | ? | ? | ? |
| Antihistamines | ? | ? | ? | ? | ? | ↑ |
| Caffeine | ↑ | ↑ | ↓ | ? | ? | ↓ |
| Alcohol | ↓ | ↑ | ↓ | ? | ↓ | ↑ |
| Cannabis | ↓ | ? | ↑ | ? | ↑ | ↑ |
| Amphetamines | ↑ | ↑ | ↓ | ↓ | ? | ↓ |

*Note.* SOL, sleep-onset latency; WASO, wake after sleep onset; TST, total sleep time; REM, rapid-eye-movement sleep; SWS, slow-wave sleep; EDS, excessive daytime somnolence. Effects: ↑ = increase; ↓ = decrease; ? = variable effects or no data.

and early-morning awakening (Mendelson, 1987). Cannabis has little effect on sleep except for an initial increase of slow-wave sleep under acute administration, followed by a decrease on recovery nights (Barratt, Beaver, & White, 1974).

Age, sleep history, circadian factors, and drugs are only a few of the many factors that can have an impact on sleep. A variety of lifestyle and behavioral variables, reviewed in later chapters, can also influence its duration and quality. Many psychological and physical conditions, as well as disorders other than insomnia (e.g., narcolepsy), may also involve sleep abnormalities. These conditions and their clinical features are reviewed in the next chapter.

## The Role and Functions of Sleep

Even after several decades of fundamental research, the exact functions of sleep remain somewhat elusive. Perhaps the only conclusion that can be drawn, based on the consistent finding that sleep deprivation leads to a natural rebound, is that sleep is necessary. Several theories ranging from evolutionary to adaptive to protective ones have postulated a variety of roles assumed by sleep (Horne, 1985, 1988b; Webb, 1979, 1988). The most parsimonious one supported by empirical evidence is that sleep serves a restorative function— physiological and psychological. Evidence from sleep deprivation experiments indicate that NREM sleep contributes primarily to restoring physical energy, whereas REM sleep plays a greater role in cognitive functions. For example, selective deprivation of slow-wave sleep (stages 3–4) leads to complaints of aching muscles and stiffness upon morning awakening. Combined with the fact that deep sleep is increased after strenuous exercise, this suggests that NREM sleep is involved in restoring physical energy (Horne, 1981; Torsvall, 1981). On the other hand, selective deprivation of REM sleep interferes with memory consolidation, thus giving REM sleep a functional role in retention of newly learned materials during wakefulness (Grosvenor & Lack, 1984; Smith & Lapp, 1991).

How much sleep do we need? The average sleep duration for adults with no sleep complaints is between 7 and 8.5 hours per night and it seems to be normally distributed (Kripke et al., 1979). There are, however, individual differences in sleep needs, as noted in Chapter 1. Some people function with as few as 4–5 hours per night, while others require 9–10 hours. There are no normative data, comparable to a table of ideal body weight for height and sex, dictating optimal sleep length. Yet sleep duration correlates with life expectancy and psychological well-being. A survey of the health and lifestyle of over 1 million persons suggests that sleep length correlates with longevity (Kripke et al., 1979). The longest life expectancy is associated with sleep durations between 7 and 7.9 hours. People who sleep for a significantly shorter duration (4 hours) or a longer duration (10 hours) have a higher incidence of heart diseases and strokes. These results, however, are strictly correlational and do not imply causality. Psychological differences between short and long sleepers have been inconsistent. Early research suggested that people whose natural tendency is to need little sleep are more active, more energetic, and better adjusted socially, whereas natural long sleepers are nonconformists and worriers (Hartmann, 1973). More recent findings, however, have failed to replicate these findings or to find any personality difference between short and long sleepers on measures of neuroticism and introversion–extraversion (Buela-Casal, Sierra, & Caballo, 1992).

## Consequences of Sleep Deprivation

The main consequences of sleep deprivation in otherwise normal sleepers are sleepiness, performance impairment, and mood alterations (Horne, 1985; Johnson, 1982). The severity of these effects depends upon whether sleep loss is partial, total, acute, or chronic. Acute sleep loss (i.e., one night) causes fatigue and decreases motivation and initiative. It has little effect on next-day performance, particularly when simple motor tasks are involved. Creativity, however, is diminished after one night of sleep loss. Impairments have been found in cognitive flexibility, the ability to change strategy, originality, and generation of unusual ideas (Horne, 1988a).

Total sleep loss for more than one night leads to microsleep episodes' intruding into wakefulness. Consequently, attention span is reduced, concentration is more difficult, and performance efficiency is impaired. As sleep loss accumulates, daytime sleepiness increases, and both cognitive and behavioral deficits are exacerbated. Studies of army personnel have shown that perception, judgment, and reaction time become particularly impaired under prolonged sleep loss conditions (see Johnson, 1982; Parkes, 1985). Mood disturbances (e.g., irritability, hostility) may occur after temporary or prolonged sleep loss. Paradoxically, sleep deprivation may have a transient antidepressant effect in some patients with endogenous depression (Gillin, 1983). The few studies reporting major personality changes have generally failed to measure premorbid status before sleep deprivation experiments. There is no known major change in biochemical or metabolic activity resulting solely from temporary sleep deprivation (Horne, 1978). Despite the commonly held belief that sleep loss lowers immune functions and increases vulnerability to certain physical ailments, there is little, if any, empirical evidence supporting this view.

The focus of recent research has switched from studying the effects of experimental sleep deprivation to that of examining the clinical impact of various sleep disorders, such as sleep apnea, periodic limb movements, and narcolepsy. The most common consequences of these disorders are nocturnal sleep fragmentation and excessive daytime sleepiness. The consequences are serious (e.g., falling asleep at the wheel), may interfere with social and occupational functioning, and may pose serious public health and safety hazards (Mitler et al., 1988). Daytime performance of individuals with these disorders is generally more impaired than that of chronic insomniacs, though the latter group is subjectively more distressed about it.

As pointed out in Chapter 1, the consequences of experimental sleep deprivation must be distinguished from the clinical impact of chronic insomnia. Participants in sleep deprivation experiments are often good sleepers to begin with, and sleep loss is always time-limited. They are usually highly motivated and challenged by the tasks involved. Demand characteristics, cognitive sets, and motivational variables are fairly different. Because of its unpredictable and uncontrollable nature, sleep loss in chronic insomniacs is very frustrating, and emotional distress is often the main consequence. Although chronic insomniacs complain of daytime sleepiness and performance decrements, objective evidence of such deficits is more limited.

# 3

# Diagnostic Considerations

*dissimilar/diverse ingredients*

Insomnia is a heterogeneous complaint with multiple origins. As basic knowledge about sleep has accumulated over the past few decades, so has our understanding of its disorders. No fewer than 88 sleep–wake disorders are described in the *International Classification of Sleep Disorders* (ICSD; ASDA, 1990). The differential diagnosis of insomnia has also become more sophisticated, and several subtypes reflecting various etiologies have been identified. What used to be considered a simple symptom of psychiatric or medical illnesses is now, in many instances, a clinical disorder in its own right. This chapter discusses the various conditions producing a complaint of insomnia. After a brief comment on nosological classification, the main insomnia subtypes, their clinical features, and etiological factors are reviewed.

*list of diseases*

## Nosological Classification

There are currently three separate nosological classifications of sleep disorders: DSM-IV (APA, in press), the 10th edition of the *International Classification of Diseases* (ICD-10; World Health Organization, 1993), and ICSD (ASDA, 1990). Although these nosologies are not always compatible with each other, most of them recognize several broad complaints or symptoms associated with the various sleep disorders. These include insomnias, hypersomnias, and parasomnias (e.g., nightmares, sleepwalking). Sleep–wake schedule disorders (e.g., jet lag, shift work) are usually classified into a separate category (i.e., circadian rhythm disorders), even though they may give rise to either insomnia or hypersomnia.

The DSM taxonomy lumps various conditions into a few clusters, emphasizing the distinction between primary insomnias and insomnias secondary to mental disorders (Axis I or Axis II) or to medical conditions (Axis III). Likewise, the ICD-10 nosology classifies insomnias, according to whether they are attributable to emotional causes or to medical or neurological disorders. The ICSD nosology also distinguishes between primary and secondary insomnias, but it further classifies the primary subtypes according to their intrinsic or extrinsic nature. Psychophysiological, subjective, and idiopathic insomnias are considered intrinsic because they are assumed to be functionally autonomous. In contrast, insomnias attributable to transient stress, inadequate sleep hygiene (e.g., excessive caffeine intake), environmental factors (e.g., light, noise), or hypnotic or alcohol dependency are extrinsic, because sleep should be normalized once the external factor has been removed.

There is substantial overlap among these subtypes, and they probably fall on a continuum rather than being distinct entities (Hauri, 1983; Reynolds, Kupfer, Buysse, Coble, & Yeager, 1991). For instance, adjustment sleep disorder (extrinsic) as a result of stressful life events may evolve into psychophysiological insomnia (intrinsic) even after the instigating event has been resolved. Likewise, insomnia caused by withdrawal from or tolerance to sustained use of hypnotic medications is often exacerbated by psychological factors. Although such distinctions are useful for assessing the relative importance of various etiological factors and for treatment planning, there is currently little empirical evidence to justify all of the subtypes that have been proposed. Accordingly, the present discussion focuses on the main insomnia subtypes that are substantiated by empirical evidence.


## The Differential Diagnosis of Insomnia

A wide variety of conditions can produce a subjective complaint of insomnia. The primary insomnias include psychophysiological, subjective, and idiopathic subtypes. They have a psychological origin, and behavioral, cognitive, and physiological factors assume a predominant etiological role. Insomnia may also be associated with psychiatric, medical, pharmacological, and environmental conditions. Other sleep disorders may be the underlying cause even though insomnia is the presenting complaint. These include sleep-induced respiratory impairment (e.g., sleep apnea), sleep-related movement disorders (e.g., periodic leg movements), disorders of the sleep–wake schedule (e.g., jet lag), and the parasomnias (e.g., night terrors). Table 3.1 lists the various insomnia conditions presented in the ICSD (ASDA, 1990). This is a slightly modified and updated version of the "disorders of initiating and maintaining sleep" published in the original *Diagnostic Classification of Sleep and Arousal Disorders* (Association of Sleep Disorders Centers, 1979).

TABLE 3.1. Primary and Secondary Insomnia Subtypes

---

*Primary insomnias*
  Psychophysiological insomnia
  Subjective insomnia (sleep state misperception)
  Idiopathic insomnia (childhood onset)
*Secondary insomnias*
  Insomnia associated with psychiatric disorders
  Insomnia associated with medical or central nervous system disorders
  Insomnia associated with alcohol or drug dependency
  Insomnia associated with environmental factors
  Insomnia associated with sleep-induced respiratory impairment
  Insomnia associated with movement disorders
  Insomnia associated with disorders of the sleep–wake schedule
  Insomnia associated with parasomnias

---

## Primary Insomnias

### PSYCHOPHYSIOLOGICAL INSOMNIA

Psychophysiological insomnia is a condition in which the subjective complaint of sleep-onset or sleep-maintenance insomnia is objectively corroborated by polysomnography. It is the most classic form of conditioned or learned insomnia, and the one that has been most extensively investigated in psychological research (Borkovec, 1982; Lacks & Morin, 1992). According to the ICSD nosology, its diagnostic features are as follows:

1. A complaint of insomnia combined with a complaint of decreased functioning during wakefulness.
2. Indications of learned sleep-preventing associations.
3. Evidence of increased somatized tension.
4. Polysomnographic evidence of an increased sleep latency, reduced sleep efficiency, and/or an increased number and duration of awakenings.
5. No evidence of other medical or psychiatric disorders that would account for the sleep disturbance.

These criteria are more clinical than operational; for this reason, the diagnosis of psychophysiological insomnia is often based on history and is only made after all other possible causes have been ruled out. This subtype of insomnia is assumed to develop as the result of two mutually reinforcing factors: learned sleep-preventing associations and somatized tension (Hauri & Fisher, 1986). The first factor stems from the conditioning taking place between sleeplessness and the stimuli normally conducive to sleep. For instance, repeated associations of disturbed sleep with situational (bed/bedroom), temporal (bedtime), or behavioral (bedtime rituals) stimuli lead to a conditioned arousal that is incompatible with sleep. This conditioning is generally implied when individuals report sleeping significantly better away from home—for example, when patients undergo a sleep laboratory evaluation and, to their surprise, wake up in the morning stating that their sleep was much better than it usually is at home. This phenomenon is also known as the "reverse first-night effect," because good sleepers typically sleep worse in a strange environment (Hauri & Olmstead, 1989). Reports from patients that they can fall asleep more easily when they do not try to (e.g., while watching TV or reading) is also used as evidence that conditioning factors are involved. Apprehension or fear of being unable to sleep often leads to performance anxiety, in which the more one strives to sleep, the less control one is able to achieve. The second factor, somatized tension, is presumed to arise from internalization of psychological conflicts; these are discharged into physiological channels, thereby leading to hyperarousal and insomnia (A. Kales & Kales, 1984). It is postulated that insomniacs focus exclusively on their sleeplessness and minimize the role other personal problems may play in their sleep disturbances.

The exact prevalence of pure psychophysiological insomnia is unclear, though a psychophysiological component is probably involved in almost all cases of chronic sleep disturbances. In our case series of 100 patients, 56% met criteria for psychophysiological insomnia as either a primary or a secondary diagnosis (Morin, Stone, et al., 1992). Although by definition psychophysiological insomniacs do not present with concurrent major psychopathology, features of both anxious and dysphoric moods are highly prevalent (Hauri & Fisher, 1986; Reynolds et al., 1984). These mood disturbances are specific to the loss of control over sleep and the impact of insomnia on daytime functioning.

Psychophysiological insomnia does not develop overnight. It is almost always preceded by situational or transient insomnia—that is, adjustment sleep disorder (ASDA, 1990), which develops in response to stressful life events. The changes in sleep patterns are temporally linked to an identifiable stressor (e.g., death of a loved one, family or marital conflicts, change of jobs, upcoming surgery). Adjustment sleep disorder is the most classic representation of the effect of psychological factors on sleep patterns. It is also the most common form of insomnia, affecting perhaps everyone at one time or another in life. Its duration is by definition time-limited, though many stressors are chronic. Although normal sleep usually resumes after the stressor is removed or the individual has adjusted to its permanent presence, excessive concerns over the initial sleep loss and fear of losing control over sleep processes may set the stage for a more pervasive form of insomnia.

## SLEEP STATE MISPERCEPTION

Also called "subjective insomnia," "pseudoinsomnia," or "experiential insomnia," sleep state misperception is a condition in which the patient's complaint of poor sleep is not corroborated by polysomnographic recordings. Despite a convincing and honest complaint of poor sleep, and no evidence of psychopathology or malingering, there is a marked discrepancy between subjective and objective sleep measures. Unlike the "reverse first-night effect" sometimes seen in psychophysiological insomnia, subjective insomniacs typically claim that their sleep is disturbed as usual when they undergo an overnight laboratory evaluation. Even in the absence of objective sleep disturbances, this subgroup seems to experience more severe daytime sequelae than does the psychophysiological subgroup (Sugerman et al., 1985).

Subjective insomniacs constitute about 5–10% of all insomniacs (Coleman et al., 1982; Trinder, 1988; Zorick, Roth, Hartse, Piccione, & Stepanski, 1981). This is perhaps the most puzzling and challenging insomnia subtype for sleep experts. This condition is still poorly understood, and there is controversy as to whether it should even be a separate diagnostic entity (McCall & Edinger, 1992; Trinder, 1988). Current EEG technology may not be sensitive enough to detect subtle brain wave patterns typical of wakefulness but scored as sleep. The standard time unit (30-second epoch) for scoring sleep stages fails to take into account momentary stage shifts occurring within a single interval. This may account for the subjective sense of continual wakefulness in patients experiencing frequent stage shifts prior to achieving persistent sleep.

Sewitch (1984) has shown that the perception of having slept is more dependent on the continuity of NREM sleep than on the actual sleep stages or sleep duration. Hauri and Olmstead (1983) also argue that EEG scoring criteria, which were initially validated against subjective and behavioral correlates, fail to take into consideration differences between good and poor sleepers in sleep perceptions. They have shown that the best match between subjective and objective measures of sleep-onset latency in insomniacs is obtained when sleep onset is defined as the first epoch of stage 2 sleep that is followed by 15 minutes of uninterrupted sleep. Several studies have also shown that the phenomenology of sleep is affected by the quantity and affective tone of the information being processed by the individual during the early sleep period (Borkovec et al., 1981; Coates et al., 1983; Gross &

Borkovec, 1982). These studies are reviewed in more detail in the next chapter.

Until further research is conducted, it would be a mistake for the clinician to assume that these patients are simply exaggerating their sleep problems. The subjective complaint of poor sleep remains a cardinal feature of all insomnias; the tendency to overestimate sleep-onset latency and to underestimate sleep duration is common among all insomniacs (Carskadon et al., 1976; Coates et al., 1982; Frankel, Coursey, Buchbinder, & Snyder, 1976), but the magnitude of these discrepancies is significantly higher among this subgroup. Perhaps individuals with true sleep state misperception represent the extreme of the continuum. Some researchers have suggested that sleep state misperception may represent the prodromic stage of psychophysiological insomnia (Salin-Pascual, Roehrs, Merlotti, Zorick, & Roth, 1992).

*precursor, before*
*running*

## IDIOPATHIC INSOMNIA

Childhood-onset or idiopathic insomnia is a lifelong inability to obtain adequate sleep (Hauri & Olmstead, 1980). It is one of the most persistent forms of insomnia and does not present the temporal fluctuations observed in psychophysiological insomnia. This condition is usually not linked to early psychological trauma or medical problems, though these factors can exacerbate the sleep disturbances. Idiopathic insomnia presumably results from an abnormality of the neurological mechanisms controlling the basic sleep-wake system. This hypothesis stems from the observation that individuals with this condition have a higher incidence of concurrent diagnoses of minimal brain dysfuctions (e.g., attention deficit disorder or dyslexia) during childhood and adolescence. Among adults, it may be accompanied by attention, concentration, memory, and motivational problems often impairing occupational functioning. Compared to psychophysiological insomniacs, idiopathic insomniacs tend to minimize the impact of disturbed sleep on their lives and display less psychological distress, even though their sleep is objectively more impaired (Hauri, 1983). They have often learned to cope early in life with chronic sleep difficulties.

Psychophysiological, subjective, and idiopathic insomnias are considered primary and intrinsic in nature. They can be further complicated by extrinsic factors, such as stress, inadequate sleep hygiene, poor sleep habits, medication, and so on. Although the ICSD describes additional insomnia subtypes based on these factors, there is extensive overlap among these conditions, and for the most part there are no empirical data to substantiate these distinct categories. Furthermore, there is no evidence to suggest differential treatment response among these subgroups. For now, I turn to those conditions initially presenting as insomnia but reflecting the presence of an underlying psychiatric, medical, pharmacological, or environmental condition or of an underlying primary sleep disorder (i.e., secondary insomnias).

## Secondary Insomnias

### INSOMNIA ASSOCIATED WITH PSYCHIATRIC DISORDERS

Sleep disturbance is a clinical feature of or a diagnostic criterion for several forms of psychopathology. Over 75% of psychiatric patients have sleep difficulties during the acute phase of their illness (Sweetwood, Grant, Kripke, Gerst, & Yager, 1980). With the exception of simple phobias, almost all anxiety conditions, especially generalized anxiety disorder, are associated with difficulties in initiating and maintaining sleep (Rosa et al., 1983; Reynolds et al., 1983; Walsh & Sugerman, 1989). Patients with nocturnal panic attacks have longer sleep-onset latency and lower sleep efficiency than normal controls (Hauri, Friedman, & Ravaris, 1989; Mellman & Unde, 1989). Night terrors or nightmares are hallmark features of post-traumatic stress disorder (Ross, Ball, Sullivan, & Caroff, 1989). Frequent and prolonged sleep interruptions, early-morning awakenings, and alterations of REM sleep are common features in dysthymia and unipolar depression (Reynolds & Kupfer, 1987; Reynolds et al., 1984). In bipolar disorder, insomnia is part of the manic phase, whereas hypersomnia is more frequent during the depressive cycle. In psychosis and dementia, the sleep–wake cycle is often reversed or delayed. Nocturnal sleep is frequently interrupted, and daytime wakefulness is compromised by frequent episodes of intruding sleep. Collectively, these findings indicate that insomnia and other sleep disorders are extremely common in patients with major psychopathology.

The incidence of psychopathology among insomniacs is higher than in good sleepers, though precise estimates vary widely depending upon the diagnostic criteria and the particular samples selected. For examples, some studies (A. Kales, Caldwell, et al., 1983) have relied on a single MMPI scale elevation (i.e., T-score above 70) as evidence of major psychopathology, while others (Jacobs, Reynolds, Kupfer, Lovin, & Ehrenpreis, 1988) have used more stringent criteria (i.e., the Research Diagnostic Criteria). Some estimates are also inflated because they are based on samples of psychiatric patients to begin with. Affective, anxiety, and substance abuse disorders are the three most prevalent Axis I diagnoses among insomniacs (Coleman et al., 1982; Ford & Kamerow, 1989; Jacobs et al., 1988; A. Kales, Caldwell, et al., 1983; Mellinger et al., 1985; Tan, Kales, Kales, Soldatos, & Bixler, 1984). Approximately 25% of insomniacs have an affective disorder, and dysthymia is the most frequent one. A similar proportion presents with anxiety-based disorders; of these, generalized anxiety disorder is the most common. Ten to fifteen percent of insomniacs have a substance abuse problem involving alcohol, sedative–hypnotics, or stimulant drugs. Adjustment and somatoform disorders are also common, though their relative prevalence is unknown. The most common Axis II diagnoses are obsessive compulsive and borderline personality disorders (Tan et al., 1984). Although these prevalence estimates suggest that most insomniacs have an underlying psychiatric disorder, there is a relatively high co-occurrence among some of those conditions (e.g., anxiety and depression). Accordingly, the best estimates currently available indicate that 35–40% of those with a primary complaint of insomnia also have one or more diagnosable psychiatric disorders.

In a survey of 100 consecutive hospitalized patients referred for a psychiatric consultation (Berlin et al., 1984), 72% complained of insomnia. All but one patient was diagnosed with transient or situational insomnia. Adjustment disorder was the most frequently associated psychiatric diagnosis ($n = 32$), followed by affective disorder ($n = 21$) and a diagnosis of "psychological factors affecting physical condition" ($n = 12$). However, there was no difference in the prevalence of psychiatric diagnoses between patients with and patients without insomnia. The factors that contributed most to the insomnia complaint were medication side effects ($n = 49$); depressed ($n = 35$) and anxious ($n = 27$) mood; pain ($n = 21$); other physical factors ($n = 10$); substance use ($n = 9$); and environmental disturbance ($n = 2$).

There is a positive relationship between the degree of psychopathology and the severity of sleep disturbances (A. Kales et al., 1984) though not all studies have confirmed this relationship (Shealy et al., 1980). In an 18-month prospective study assessing the time course of sleep disturbance in psychiatric patients and normal controls, the severity and chronicity of insomnia were positively related to the intensity of psychiatric symptomatology but not to specific diagnoses (Sweetwood et al., 1980). The relative date of onset of both conditions, however, was not reported, leaving the issue of what is cause and what is consequence unanswered. Other longitudinal data have in fact suggested that chronic insomnia may increase the vulnerability to future major depression (Ford & Kamerow, 1989). To clarify these issues, it will be essential in future studies to determine whether depression followed or predated the onset of insomnia.

In summary, comorbidity between sleep and psychological disturbances is extremely prevalent. The direction of the relationship between these conditions is often equivocal. More than 75% of psychiatric patients complain of significant sleep disturbances, whereas about 35% of those with a primary complaint of insomnia meet criteria for concurrent psychopathology. Although psychological distress is a frequent concomitant of chronic insomnia, it does not necessarily mean psychopathology, and distress specifically resulting from chronic sleep difficulties must be distinguished from that associated with psychiatric disorders. For some conditions (e.g., psychosis, major depression), it is relatively easy to establish that disturbed sleep is only one of several symptoms of the underlying psychiatric disorder. For less severe conditions, however, it is almost impossible to determine whether psychological distress is the cause or the consequence of sleep disturbances. Longitudinal studies monitoring the onset and temporal course of these two parameters are needed to clarify these issues. Meanwhile, the sole presence of psychological distress or minor psychopathology should not preclude treatment specifically targeting the sleep complaints (Morin, Kowatch, & O'Shanick, 1990; Tan et al., 1987).

## INSOMNIA ASSOCIATED WITH MEDICAL FACTORS

Acute and chronic medical illnesses can cause sleep disturbances, as a result of either their underlying symptoms or the medications or procedures used to alleviate these symptoms (Erman, 1987; Mitler et al., 1991). Almost any condition producing pain or physical discomfort is likely to cause insomnia. Disturbed sleep is often the first effect of acute pain and one of the most disabling sequelae of chronic pain (Follick, Smith, & Ahern, 1985). It is particularly frequent in patients with low back pain, arthritis, osteoporosis, headaches, and cancer (Atkinson, Ancoli-Israel, Slater, Garfin, & Gillin, 1988; Pilowsky, Crettenden, & Townley, 1985; Wittig, Zorick, Blumer, Heilbroon, & Roth, 1982). Complaints of interrupted and unrefreshing sleep combined with early-morning stiffness and daytime fatigue are extremely common in those with musculoskeletal pain. These complaints are often associated with alpha–delta sleep (i.e., frequent intrusion of alpha rhythms [wakefulness] into NREM sleep), which is subjectively experienced as a state of wakefulness continually intruding into sleep (Moldofsky, 1989; Saskin, Moldofsky, & Lue, 1986).

Congestive heart failures and chronic pulmonary diseases are almost always associated with sleep disturbances (Williams, 1988; Wooten, 1989). Endocrine (hyperthyroidism) and gastrointestinal (reflux) diseases can also interfere with sleep initiation or maintenance. In renal diseases, poor blood circulation of the extremities is associated with restless legs and periodic limb movements, leading, respectively, to sleep-onset and sleep-maintenance insomnia. Most central nervous system disorders cause severe sleep difficulty, and with advanced neurological deterioration, sleep stages become more difficult to distinguish. Disorders of the circadian rhythm are also common. The "sundown syndrome" in Alzheimer's disease, characterized by nocturnal wandering and confusion, is a major concern for caregivers and often leads to institutionalization. Almost any form of brain insult disturbs the sleep–wake cycle, often causing insomnia at night and hypersomnia during the day (Kowatch, 1989). The severity of these disturbances is proportional to the extent of the head injury, with brainstem lesions producing significantly more alteration of the sleep–wake cycle than closed head injuries. In chronic illnesses, psychological, behavioral, and lifestyle factors often exacerbate sleep problems, and these factors may require therapeutic attention in themselves.

Insomnia is often a direct side effect of medications prescribed for physical illnesses. In one study of hospitalized patients, this factor alone was implicated in over 68% of insomnia complaints (Berlin et al., 1984). In another study (Gislason & Almqvist, 1987), chronic pulmonary disease patients treated pharmacologically (with bronchodilators) were twice as likely to have sleep disturbances as those untreated or those treated with other medications. Steroids, thyroid preparations, bronchodilators, and some anti-hypertensive medications (including beta-blockers such as propranolol) and diuretics can all cause insomnia (see Chapter 2).

## INSOMNIA ASSOCIATED WITH ALCOHOL OR DRUG DEPENDENCY

Insomnia associated with drug or alcohol dependency is characterized by almost daily use of a sleep-promoting agent for at least 3 weeks (ASDA, 1990). Long-term use of most hypnotics leads to tolerance and to a corresponding decrease of the sleep-inducing effects. Increased dosage may temporarily prolong effectiveness, but daytime residual effects become more severe. Abrupt withdrawal from the medications produces a worsening of sleep difficulties above and beyond baseline levels (Gillin et al., 1989). In turn, this reinforces the insomniac's belief that medication is needed, and it perpetuates the drug dependency cycle. Alcohol-dependent insomnia is characterized by the almost nightly use of ethanol as a sleeping aid. This condition is distinguished from the typical alcoholic drinking patterns, in that drinking is limited to the 3–4 hours preceding bedtime and apparently does not interfere with social and occupational functioning. When used as a sleep-inducing substance, cannabis may produce a similar dependence. Some people self-medicate with various over-the-counter sleep aids. Not only is their clinical impact on sleep doubtful (J. D. Kales, Tan, Swearingen, & Kales, 1971), but sometimes these agents are used strictly on a prophylactic basis. Some individuals remain on low doses of benzodiazepines for years despite a complete loss of hypnotic effects (Schneider-Helmert, 1988). As such, drug-dependent insomnia is often more psychological than physical in nature.

Although sleep may normalize after a sustained drug-free period, sometimes it remains disturbed for prolonged periods, prompting individuals to resume usage of these sleep-promoting agents. The prevalence of drug-dependent insomnia is about 10–15%. Of those seeking treatment in our clinic, however, more than 50% present with a self-controlled yet habitual pattern of drug use. The management of this condition is addressed in Chapter 11.

## INSOMNIA ASSOCIATED WITH ENVIRONMENTAL FACTORS

Various environmental conditions can result in insomnia: light, noise, heat, cold, an uncomfortable mattress, or movements of a bed partner. The need to remain alert in a situation of danger, or to provide care to an infant or to an ill significant other, can also interfere with sleep. These environmental factors almost always result in sleep disturbances, though some people can also sleep under almost any environmental conditions. In those with this type of insomnia, there is a direct temporal relationship between the onset, time course, and termination of the sleep problem and the presumed causative environmental condition. Insomnia in hospitalized patients is perhaps the most common example of environmentally induced insomnia. Excessive noise and lighting conditions and the need to undergo medical procedures can disrupt sleep even in those who usually have no insomnia problem. The physical rather than psychological properties of the environmental factor presumably lead to disturbed sleep, though these two factors are rarely exclusive of each other.

## INSOMNIA ASSOCIATED WITH OTHER SLEEP DISORDERS

Several sleep disorders can produce a subjective complaint of insomnia. Polysomnography is essential to diagnose most of these conditions. I review in this section the clinical features and symptoms of sleep disorders that may initially present as insomnia.

*Sleep Apnea.* Sleep apnea is a breathing disorder in which respiration is impaired during sleep but normal during wakefulness (Guilleminault, 1989). An "apnea" is defined as a cessation of airflow at the mouth and nostrils for at least 10 seconds; a "hypopnea" involves a decrease rather than a complete cessation of airflow. There are three types of apneas: obstructive, central, and mixed. In obstructive apnea, thoracic and abdominal respiratory efforts persist in the absence of effective airflow. In central apnea, airflow and respiratory movements temporarily cease because of disordered neurological regulation of respiration. Mixed apneas begin with a central component and end with an obstructive one. The typical sequence of events involves cessation of brea- thing, arousal, resumption of breathing characteristically associated with snorting and gasping sounds, and return to sleep (Kwentus, Schultz, Fairman, & Isrow, 1985). In severe cases, this cycle may repeat itself 200–300 times a night, unbeknownst to the patient. These disordered breathing events are typically witnessed by a bedmate.

The main symptoms of apnea are snoring, pauses in breathing during sleep, restless sleep, and excessive daytime sleepiness. The condition is particularly prevalent in obese middle-aged males. Although most people experience a few apneic events, the clinical significance of apnea is determined by the frequency and duration of respiratory disturbances and by other complications. Apneic events are usually associated with arousals, hypoxemia, and cardiac arrhythmias. Neuropsychological deficits, such as memory and concentration problems, are also common (Bédard, Montplaisir, Richer, Rouleau, & Malo, 1991; Greenberg, Watson, & Deptula, 1987; Stone et al., 1992); however, it is still unclear whether these deficits are attributable to hypoxemia, sleep fragmentation, or a combination of both factors (Bliwise, 1989). The most direct consequence of sleep apnea is chronic sleep fragmentation, which leads to difficulty in staying awake during the day. Because patients who suffer from this condition are usually unaware of the nocturnal symptoms, the only subjective complaint is often one of daytime sleepiness. In some cases, however, prolonged respiratory disturbances may lead a person to wake up gasping for air and experiencing panic-like attacks, with ensuing difficulty in returning to sleep. Thus, although excessive daytime sleepiness is a much more frequent complaint, sleep maintenance insomnia may also be the presenting complaint, especially in patients with central apnea.

*Restless-Legs Syndrome.* Restless-legs syndrome is diagnosed on a clinical basis and is described as an uncomfortable aching sensation in the calves, accompanied by an irresistible urge to move the legs. It may also involve the thighs, the feet, the knees, and even the arms. Walking or stretching of the legs can alleviate this unpleasant sensation. Restless legs is experienced during wakefulness, but is typically worse at bedtime. It can considerably delay sleep onset and may be the primary cause of sleep-onset insomnia. Restless legs must be differentiated from a generalized bodily restlessness seen in anxious insomniacs. Most individuals with restless-legs syndrome also present with periodic limb movements during sleep.

*Periodic Limb Movements.* Periodic limb movements consist of brief (lasting 0.5–5 seconds), repetitive (occurring every 20–40 seconds), and highly stereotyped movements of the limbs (legs and arms) occurring during sleep (Montplaisir & Godbout, 1989). They are more frequent in the first third of the night. They are often associated with arousals, but not necessarily with full awakenings; consequently, the patient is unaware of these movements.

Occasionally, an individual may wake up with leg cramps, though a spouse is usually the one noticing these movements. This disorder must be distinguished from the "hypnic jerk" occuring at sleep onset or from phasic limb twitches of REM sleep, both of which are normal phenomena. The prevalence of periodic limb movements, also called "nocturnal myoclonus," increases significantly with aging (Ancoli-Israel, Kripke, Mason, & Kaplan, 1985). It is frequently associated with chronic pain (particularly when the pain radiates down to the lower extremities), with renal diseases, and with other medical conditions causing poor blood circulation (e.g., diabetes). The subjective complaint associated with periodic limb movements is either sleep-maintenance insomnia or excessive daytime sleepiness. However, patients are sometimes totally asymptomatic, and the clinical significance of periodic limb movements in these individuals is unclear.

*Circadian Rhythm Disorders.* Circadian rhythm disorders are dysfunctions related to the timing of the major sleep episode within the 24-hour day. The main clinical feature shared by these disorders is a misalignment between the individual sleep–wake schedule and that which is desired or regarded as the societal norm (ASDA, 1990). The resulting complaint is that the individual cannot either sleep or stay awake when he or she wishes or needs to do so. Examples of circadian rhythm disorders that may present as insomnia include conditions associated with rapid time zone changes (jet lag), night or shift work, and phase-delay and phase-advance syndromes. These disorders share a chronobiological basis, which can be either intrinsic or extrinsic in nature. For example, phase-delay syndrome presumably has an internal chronobiological basis, whereas disorders resulting from a rotating or night shift are generally caused by scheduling factors imposed by societal or occupational obligations.

In phase-delay syndrome, the major sleep period is delayed in relation to its desired timing. It is characterized by intractable difficulty in falling asleep until late in the night (e.g., 3:00 A.M.). Consequently, arising at a conventional time in the morning to fulfill occupational obligations is extremely difficult because of the protracted duration of the previous sleep period. There is usually no difficulty in staying asleep once sleep has been achieved (Weitzman et al., 1981). Accordingly, when there is no required arising time, such as on weekends or during vacations, the problem may be alleviated by the normal sleep duration (despite its delayed nature). College students and people working night or rotating shifts are more likely to develop this disorder. Irregular sleep schedules, or frequent switches in bedtimes and arising times, tend to desynchronize the circadian rhythms and predispose individuals to a phase-delay problem. This condition is to be distinguished from psychophysiological insomnia and may require a different intervention. Chronotherapy and light therapy have been used for resetting the circadian rhythm in such cases (Czeisler et al., 1981; Rosenberg, 1991).

In the phase-advance syndrome, the presenting complaint involves a compelling difficulty in staying awake during the evening, followed by early-morning awakening. Total sleep duration is not shortened. The notion of control is important in evaluating this condition. Individuals with this problem do not choose to go to bed early in the evening; they are simply unable to remain awake until their desired bedtime. More frequent in older adults, the phase-advance syndrome must be differentiated from early-morning awakening, which is also a common form of sleep-maintenance insomnia in late life. Difficulty in staying awake after 8:00 or 9:00 in the evening, followed by early awakening (e.g., 4:00 the next morning), may reflect a phase-advance sleep disorder instead of a true sleep-maintenance problem. In making a differential diagnosis, the clinician should always consider the duration of the previous sleep episode instead of relying exclusively on the actual clock time of the final awakening.

*Parasomnias.* Parasomnias are disorders of arousal, disorders of sleep–wake transition, or dysfunctions occurring primarily in REM sleep. They represent abnormal or excessive activation of the central nervous system, involving changes in autonomic or skeletal muscle activity. Rhythmic movement disorders (e.g., head banging, body rocking) typically occur during the transitional period from wakefulness to sleep. Somnambulism (sleepwalking) and night terrors are arousal disorders occurring during stages 3–4 sleep, whereas nightmares originate from REM sleep (Nino-Murcia & Dement, 1987). Much more frequent during childhood, those conditions are usually outgrown by late adolescence. Parasomnias do not necessarily lead to a complaint of insomnia or hypersomnia, though in the most severe forms either of these difficulties may be present. In many cases, they are simply undesirable phenomena. However, some parasomnias may cause physical injuries (REM behavior disorder, sleepwalking) and significant psychological distress (night terror) to patients, spouses, or caregivers (Nino-Murcia & Dement, 1987; Schenck, Milner, Hurwitz, Bundlie, & Mahowald, 1989).

## Conclusion

Numerous potential factors may give rise to a subjective complaint of insomnia. Psychological, medical, pharmacological, and environmental factors must be considered; even when these have been ruled out, another sleep disorder (e.g., apnea) may still be the underlying cause of insomnia. The diagnosis of a primary insomnia is often made by exclusion. There is extensive overlap among the various primary insomnia subtypes, and these conditions probably fall on a continuum rather than being distinct entities. Although treatment should focus on the underlying causes, behavioral and cognitive factors are almost always implicated in exacerbating chronic insomnia. The intervention described in this book is designed not only for pure cases of primary insomnias, but for a heterogeneous subset of patients with or without associated psychological, medical, and substance abuse problems.

# 4

---

# A Cognitive-Behavioral
# Conceptualization of Insomnia

Various diagnostic subtypes of insomnia, along with their clinical features and presumed causes, have been described in the preceding chapter. This chapter provides a more focused view of psychological factors implicated in the mediation of primary insomnias. Several hypotheses that emphasize different but complementary causative factors are summarized. An integrative model addressing temporal, environmental, and organismic variables is presented. This conceptual framework sets the foundations for the treatment protocol described in subsequent chapters. I begin by outlining a conceptual model of the natural evolution of insomnia over time in terms of common predisposing traits, precipitating events, and perpetuating conditions.

## The Natural History of Insomnia

To various degrees, everyone is predisposed to develop sleep disturbances. Although some people never exceed the insomnia threshold, many will at some point in their lives experience sleepless nights. Sleep is very sensitive to psychological and physical ailments, so acute insomnia is generally precipitated by emotional life stressors or by health-related factors. Most individuals resume their normal sleep patterns after a precipitating event has abated, or after they have adjusted to its permanent presence, but others continue to suffer persistent insomnia long after these instigating factors are removed. Figure 4.1 depicts a conceptual model of how insomnia evolves over time from a situational problem to a chronic one.

According to Spielman (Spielman, 1986; Spielman & Glovinsky, 1991), three types of factors operate in the natural history of insomnia: (1) predisposing conditions, or enduring traits that lower the threshold needed for triggering insomnia; (2) precipitating circumstances, or the temporal and contextual factors surrounding the onset of insomnia; and (3) the perpetuating factors, or

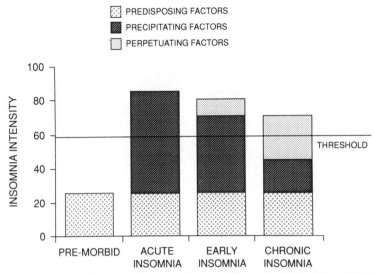

FIGURE 4.1. The natural history of insomnia. From Spielman, A., & Glovinsky, P. (1991). The varied nature of insomnia. In P. J. Hauri (Ed.), *Case studies in insomnia* (pp. 1–15). New York: Plenum Press. Copyright 1991 by Plenum Publishing Corporation. Reprinted by permission of the publisher and authors.

those variables contributing to the maintenance of insomnia over time. The relative importance assumed by these factors changes over time. A cardinal assumption of this model is that insomnia may become independent of or functionally autonomous from its origins. Regardless of the nature of the precipitating events, additional controlling variables are superimposed on these factors in maintaining the sleep problem. Treatment should then focus on these perpetuating factors, even though the former conditions may still be instrumental in maintaining sleep difficulties.

## Predisposing Factors

Several predisposing factors may increase the vulnerability of some individuals to exceed a critical threshold needed to develop insomnia. The construct of arousability is a core mediating feature of insomnia. Coren (1988) conceptualizes arousability as a relatively stable predisposition that manifests itself not only in the predorminal phase but as a permanent behavioral trait. It can be expressed as physiological, cognitive, or emotional hyperarousal (Espie, 1991; A. Kales & Kales, 1984; Lacks, 1987). Insomniacs are more physiologically aroused than good sleepers, not only at night, but during the day as well. Their cognitive style is often characterized as obsessive, worrisome, hypervigilant, and anxiety-prone. Although not all insomniacs fit this profile, some tend to internalize emotional conflicts and channel this into physiological arousal (A. Kales & Kales, 1984). Most forms of psychopathology, particularly affective and anxiety disorders, increase the vulnerability to sleep disturbances. On the other hand, hyperarousal has been implicated in several forms of psychopathology; it may be a common thread in some clinical dysfunctions, not a unique characteristic of insomnia. In addition, although the role of arousal in mediating insomnia is relatively clear, what is less certain is whether this is a state or a trait. The lack of longitudinal studies precludes the assumption that hyperarousal predates the onset of insomnia. Chronically disturbed sleep may lead to excessive arousal as well.

A large proportion of our clinical patients report that at least one family member also experiences insomnia. Coren and Searleman (1985) found that more than 75% of sampled college students whose mothers reported disrupted sleep patterns also had problems initiating or maintaining sleep. These observations indicate that insomnia runs in families, but it is unclear whether this reflects a genetic predisposition (Heath, Kendler, Eaves, & Martin, 1990) or whether poor sleep habits are learned through parental modeling influences. The co-occurrence of minimal brain dysfunctions (e.g., learning disabilities, attention deficit disorders) with childhood-onset insomnia suggests that some individuals may inherently be more predisposed to sleep disturbances, owing, perhaps, to a deficiency in the basic neural mechanisms of arousal (Hauri & Olmstead, 1983).

Insomnia is twice as common in women as in men, and, as such, female gender may be a risk factor. Age-related factors may also increase this vulnerability. Although insomnia is not an inevitable consequence of aging, the increased incidence of health problems and medication use in late life, combined with naturally occurring changes in sleep patterns of older adults (e.g., lowered awakening threshold, decreased stages 3–4 sleep), place this segment of the population at greater risk for insomnia. Finally, a previous complaint of insomnia is apparently a risk factor for future sleep difficulties (Klink, Quan, Kaltenborn, & Lebowitz, 1992). It is important to note that there have been no prospective studies of the premorbid characteristics of persons at risk for the development of chronic insomnia (A. Kales & Vgontzas, 1992). Thus, most of the predisposing factors reviewed so far remain hypothetical, because they are based on retrospective and correlational evidence.

## Precipitating Factors

Stress is the most common precipitant of insomnia. About 74% of poor sleepers recall specific stressful life experiences associated with the onset of their insomnia, and the frequency of occurrence of such events is greater during the year the sleep problem began than in either the previous or subsequent years (Healy et al., 1981). Personal losses through separation, divorce, or the death of a loved one are those most often associated with the onset of insomnia. Family-, health-, and work-related stressors naturally lead to sleepless nights. Illnesses or hospitalization also often cause trouble sleeping; this can be the direct result of physical ailments or of concomitant emotional turmoil. Finally, chronic stress on the job or long-term conflicts with family members may not only trigger sleep problems but also exacerbate them.

The circumstances surrounding the onset of sleep difficulties are particularly relevant to the management of acute insomnia, and the most appropriate interventions usually involve correction or removal of the underlying precipitating condition. As noted earlier, most people usually resume normal sleep after a stressful life event is resolved or after they have adjusted to it. Sometimes, though, a transient sleep problem that seems to be caused by a situational stressor does not resolve itself and develops into a full-fledged case of chronic insomnia. People with a higher predisposition to begin with may be particularly vulnerable to this progressive deterioration, though there have been no longitudinal investigations of the natural history of acute insomnia and its relationship to chronic insomnia.

## Perpetuating Factors

When disturbed sleep has persisted long after the precipitating circumstances have been altered, attention should be shifted to the perpetuating conditions. Although the instigating events may be chronic in nature, the most salient conditions maintaining insomnia consist of maladaptive sleep habits and dysfunctional cognitions about sleep loss and its impact on a person's life. These factors are discussed more extensively later. For the time being, let it suffice to say that a variety of maladaptive behavior patterns often used to alleviate insomnia (e.g., hypnotic use) or to compensate for sleep loss (e.g., excessive amounts of time spent in bed, irregular sleep schedule, napping) may combine with dysfunctional, affect-laden cognitions (e.g., worry over sleep loss, rumination over daytime deficits, performance anxiety, fear of losing control, learned helplessness) and other factors (e.g., secondary gains) to perpetuate a problem that might have otherwise been only temporary.

To summarize this conceptual framework, several factors in various degrees may predispose people to developing sleep disturbances. Even though psychosocial stressors, physical illness, or other life events may have instigated insomnia initially, a variety of behavioral and cognitive factors may exacerbate the sleep problem. The original precipitating factors may continue to have a negative influence, but the main focus of treatment should be on altering or removing the maintaining conditions.

## Insomnia Etiology

Several models have been proposed to explain the etiological mechanisms of insomnia. This section reviews the main empirical findings on the role of physiological, cognitive, and emotional hyperarousal; information processing and time estimation; and conditioning. Etiological research has focused predominantly on the mechanisms interfering with sleep onset, and it is unclear whether these factors are also involved in sleep-maintenance problems.

### Physiological Arousal

Because sleep is associated with reduced autonomic activity, it is widely assumed that physiological arousal causes insomnia. Several investigations have shown that insomniacs, compared to good sleepers, have faster heart rate, more elevated frontalis muscle tension, and greater electrodermal conductance either during the presleep period, during sleep, or following nocturnal awakenings (Freedman & Sattler, 1982; Haynes, Adams, & Franzen, 1981; Haynes, Fitzgerald, Shute, & O'Meary, 1985; Monroe, 1967). Although some studies have failed to replicate these findings (Good, 1975; Gross & Borkovec, 1982), research using 24-hour monitoring of core body temperature has yielded additional support for the role of autonomic arousal. There is a close covariation between body temperature and alertness–sleepiness, with the propensity to fall asleep being greatest as temperature declines and alertness being maximal on its rising slope (Monk & Moline, 1989). Insomniacs also display higher temperature both during the day and at night than good sleepers, as well as less cyclic variation. Morris et al. (1990) documented a phase delay of almost 2.5 hours in the temperature rhythm of insomniacs, which was associated with sleep-onset difficulties. It is unclear, however, whether these data reflect a natural phase delay or are by-products of behavioral factors (e.g., irregularity of bedtimes and arising times) among insomniacs. Finally, data from the Multiple Sleep Latency Test, a measure of daytime physiological tendency, show that insomniacs are no more sleepy during the day than normal controls, despite more disrupted sleep at night (Seidel et al., 1984; Stepanski et al., 1988; Sugerman et al., 1985). Although the validity of this test with insomniacs is controversial, these findings collectively suggest that autonomic arousal interferes with the initiation and maintenance of sleep, and that insomniacs are hyperaroused not only at night but equally during the day.

These data have led to a variety of interventions aimed at lowering physiological arousal. Relaxation-based methods (e.g., progressive muscle relaxation, EMG biofeedback, autogenic training) are the most frequently used psychological interventions for insomnia. Although their clinical benefits for sleep have been extensively documented, the underlying mechanisms of such benefits are still unclear. Most studies have failed to demonstrate that lowered physiological arousal (e.g., heart rate, frontalis EMG) is paralleled by subjectively or objectively defined sleep improvements (Borkovec, 1982; Morin & Kwentus, 1988). The lack of a relationship between process (lowered autonomic activity) and outcome (improved sleep) casts some doubts on the validity of the physiological hyperarousal hypothesis, at least as a model explaining all forms of insomnia.

## Cognitive Arousal

A competing theory postulates that cognitive rather than physiological arousal causes insomnia. Cognitive arousal can be a negative, a neutral, or even a positive experience. It may be expressed in terms of worry, racing mind, rumination, intrusive thoughts, planning, analyzing, or difficulty in controlling exciting thoughts. According to this model, excessive cognitive activity, whether pleasant or not, interferes with the sleep process. A survey of causal attributions of insomnia among self-defined poor sleepers indicates that cognitive arousal is blamed 10 times more frequently (55%) than somatic arousal (5%) as its main determinant (Lichstein & Rosenthal, 1980). Over one-third (35%) of the subjects claim that both types of arousal are important factors, while 5% endorse neither component. Nicassio, Mendlowitz, Fussell, and Petras (1985) developed a two-factor scale measuring both types of presleep arousal, and also found that the cognitive factor was more strongly associated with sleep-onset insomnia than the somatic one.

Direct manipulations of cognitive intrusion have yielded additional evidence supporting the mediational role of cognitive hyperactivity. For example, a sample of good sleepers who were informed that they would have to present a speech after a daytime nap took significantly longer to fall asleep than control subjects (Gross & Borkovec, 1982). Likewise, exposure to a mild stressor (an arithmetic task) at bedtime delayed sleep onset in good sleepers but actually hastened it in insomniacs (Haynes et al., 1981). The authors suggest that exposure to a mild stressor, especially a non-sleep-related one, may counteract the already elevated rate of sleep-related cognitions among insomniacs. The process involved here is analogous to treatment methods (e.g., imagery training) aimed at controlling intrusive thoughts (Woolfolk &

McNulty, 1983), in that it disrupts the flow of negative and more affectively laden sleep cognitions (e.g., fear of sleeplessness, performance anxiety, etc.). This explanation is partly supported by other data showing that deficits of internal attentional control, which may prevent the screening out of sleep-incompatible thoughts, are associated with prolonged sleep latency in older insomniacs (Shute, Fitzgerald, & Haynes, 1986).

On the basis of Davidson's (1978) theory that activation of some physi-ological systems (e.g., skin conductance) is indicative of cognitive rather than somatic arousal, Lichstein and Fanning (1990) explored the relative role of these two factors by exposing subjects to a stressor while monitoring several physiological parameters. During baseline conditions, insomniacs displayed more variable skin conductance and higher frontalis muscle tension than did good sleepers. When exposed to the stressor (i.e., a threat of shock as a result of malfunctioning equipment), insomniacs showed more reactivity than con-trols on the skin conductance measure, which was interpreted as reflecting anxious ruminations in the former group. No such reactivity was obtained on the measure of muscle tension, which was interpreted as lack of support for the mediational role of somatic arousal.

To explore the role of cognitive arousal, several investigations have used a thought-sampling procedure during the presleep period and have examined the rate, content, and affective tone of these cognitions (Borkovec et al., 1981; Coates et al., 1983; Freedman & Sattler, 1982; Van Egeren, Haynes, Fran-zen, & Hamilton, 1983). The results relating to content and affective tone, which discriminate poor from good sleepers, are reviewed in the next section on emotional arousal. The results addressing the rate of cognitive activity alone are inconsistent. Freedman and Sattler (1982) found no difference in the level of presleep mental activity between poor and good sleepers. In contrast, other investigators (Coates et al., 1983) have indicated that excessive cognitive activity is related to degree of sleep difficulty and to discrepancies between reported and recorded sleep. Thus, it is unclear whether an excessive rate of cognitive intrusions is causing insomnia. Being awake for longer periods of time naturally provides more opportunity to think. However, there are no data showing that for the same presleep interval length (i.e., 20–30 minutes), poor sleepers process more information cognitively than good sleepers do. Thus, an important issue that remains unresolved is whether cognitive arousal is causing insomnia or whether it simply represents an epiphenomenon of wakefulness (Borkovec, 1979, 1982).

Despite some conflicting results, the overall evidence suggests that cognitive activation is involved in mediating sleep disturbances. These find-ings have led to an increasing use of treatment methods (e.g., imagery training, meditation, thought stopping, time out for worry) aimed at control-ling excessive presleep cognitive activity (Morin & Azrin, 1987, 1988; Schoicket, Bertelson, & Lacks, 1988; Woolfolk & McNulty, 1983). The relationships between treatment process (i.e., attenuation of excessive menta-tion) and outcome (e.g., reduced sleep-onset latency) have been stronger than those with somatic arousal (Mitchell, 1979; Mitchell & White, 1977; White & Nicassio, 1990; Woolfolk & McNulty, 1983), though in one study (Sana-vio, 1988) matching of subjects who displayed high levels of cognitive arousal with a cognitive intervention did not yield superior results to a mismatched condition.

## Emotional Arousal

There has been a recent shift of attention from the somatic versus cognitive dichotomy to a more direct focus on the emotional underpinning of arousal (Espie, 1991; Lacks, 1987; A. Kales & Kales, 1984). Increasing evidence indicates that the content and affective valence of cognitions (beliefs, ex-pectations, attributions) is an important mediating factor of insomnia. For example, insomniacs hold more unrealistic expectations about their sleep requirements and stronger beliefs about the consequences of insomnia than normal sleepers (Morin, Stone, Trinkle, Mercer, & Remsberg, in press). Their causal attributions tend to be more external (i.e., insomnia is believed to be the result of a biochemical imbalance) and unstable (i.e., sleep is perceived as uncontrollable and unpredictable). In turn, these dysfunctional cognitions correlate with insomnia severity and emotional distress. When the content and affective valence of insomniacs' cognitions are sampled at night, they also tend to be more negatively toned than those of good sleepers (Borkovec et al., 1981; Kuisk, Bertelson, & Walsh, 1989). Thoughts that are negative and sleep-related (e.g., thoughts about not falling asleep, fear of the consequences of sleep loss) are associated with more severe sleep difficulties (Van Egeren et al., 1983). Thus, dysfunctional beliefs and attitudes about sleep can trigger emotional arousal and feed into the insomnia problem.

Descriptive studies of the psychological profile of insomniacs have re-ported elevated measures indicative of anxiety, dysphoria, worry, somatized tension, or neuroticism in general (Edinger et al., 1988; Freedman & Sattler, 1982; Hauri & Fisher, 1986; A. Kales & Kales, 1984). In turn, this psycholog-ical makeup may heighten the affective response of insomniacs to poor sleep (Coyle & Watts, 1991) and trigger dysfunctional sleep cognitions. Thus, insomniacs tend to endorse state (presleep) and trait (daytime) measures reflecting an anxious, dysphoric, or worrisome cognitive style, and these measures correlate with sleep disruptions.

Reactivity to stress is another important variable mediating insomnia. The frequency and intensity of daytime stressors are related to difficulties in initiating (White & Nicassio, 1990) and maintaining (Rubman et al., 1990) sleep. This relationship is partly mediated by the level of arousal at bedtime.

Following exposure to stress, individuals who remain more cognitively aroused in the presleep period experience more sleep difficulties than those who are able to control their presleep arousal (White & Nicassio, 1990). Insomniacs may be more emotionally reactive to stressors and may take longer to recover from exposure to such events (Waters, Adams, Binks, & Varnado, 1993). Their coping mechanisms may also be deficient, in that they tend to internalize conflicts and ruminate about what they should have done or said in a given situation. In contrast, people who cope more adaptively with daily hassles, perhaps by communicating more assertively, go to bed with freer minds. These observations suggest that insomniacs are hypersensitive and overrespond to stimulations judged to be of minimal intensity by others.

In summary, the content and affective tone of sleep-related cognitions seem to assume a greater role in insomnia than the rate of cognitive activity alone. Exposure and reactivity to stressful events, as well as coping skills, may also influence the role of emotional arousal. These findings, combined with the increasing popularity of cognitive interventions, have naturally led to an increasing use of treatment methods targeting dysfunctional sleep cognitions (Morin & Stone, 1992; Morin, Kowatch, Barry, & Walton, 1993; Sanavio, 1988; Sanavio, Vidotto, Bettinardi, Rolletto, & Zorzi, 1990).

## Information Processing and Time Estimation

The phenomenological experience of sleep differs quantitatively and qualitatively between poor and good sleepers. For instance, when awakened from stage 2 sleep, insomniacs report being awake already more frequently than good sleepers (Borkovec et al., 1981; Coates et al., 1983). Insomniacs also overestimate sleep-onset latency and underestimate sleep duration in comparison to EEG measures (Coates et al., 1982). These discrepancies are present in all insomniacs, though their magnitude is disproportionally higher in the subjective ones. The perception of sleep–wakefulness is strongly dependent on accurate time estimation, which itself is dependent on several factors.

Research into basic information processing shows that time estimation is affected by the quantity and content of information being processed, as well as by the situational context (Fichten & Libman, 1991). In a relaxing and pleasant situation (e.g., sensory deprivation experiments), there is a tendency to underestimate duration of elapsed time. Conversely, in an aversive or unpleasant situation (e.g., lying awake in bed for an extensive period of time), the subjective perception of time seems longer than the actual "clock time" (Frankel et al., 1976). Borkovec (1982) has proposed that "distorted time perception and wake-like phenomenology during the early sleep and possibly during lighter sleep stages throughout the night" are attributable to excessive cognitive activity in insomniacs as compared to good sleepers. The perception of time seems longer as the amount of information being processed per unit of time increases. Time estimation is significantly altered in an information-processing overload condition relative to an underload condition. Accordingly, excessive cognitive activation is linked to greater discrepancies between subjective and objective measurements of sleep (Coates et al., 1983). Perceptual time distortions are even more pronounced when the affective tone of the information being processed is negative (Borkovec et al., 1981) and when the subject is an active participant rather than a mere observer of the unfolding activity (Coates et al., 1983). Worrying is also associated with cortical arousal (Carter, Johnson, & Borkovec, 1986) and creates a condition of sensory overload. The inability to control internal attentional processes may accentuate perceptual distortions (Shute et al., 1986). Finally, the sole fact of waiting for an event to occur (i.e., waiting to fall asleep) may lengthen the subjective perception of elapsed time (Fichten & Libman, 1991). Several of these issues have been nicely addressed by Fichten and Libman (1991), who recently reviewed evidence from the experimental literature on perception and sensation (Coren & Ward, 1989; Fraisse, 1984).

Collectively, these findings suggest that excessive arousal alters time estimation, which in turn affects the perception of sleep–wakefulness. These issues are particularly relevant for understanding the discrepancies between reported and recorded sleep in subjective insomnia (i.e., sleep state misperception), and may also explain similar discrepancies of a lower magnitude in psychophysiological insomniacs. Cognitive therapy and corrective feedback (Downey & Bonnet, 1992) may be instrumental in modifying these perceptual distortions.

## Conditioning Variables

Classical and operant conditioning principles play an important role in sleep induction and are equally involved in difficulties in initiating and in maintaining sleep. Animal experiments have shown that electrical stimulation of the preoptic area in the forebrain produces an EEG synchronization similar to that of sleep (see Spielman, Caruso, & Glovinsky, 1987). After repeated pairings of this unconditioned stimulus with a neutral stimulus (e.g., a tone), sleep can be induced by the sole presentation of the neutral (i.e., conditioned) stimulus. Several experiments on the phenomenon of conditioned tolerance to drugs (e.g., benzodiazepines) have also yielded strong empirical evidence to implicate conditioning factors in insomnia (King, Bouton, & Musty, 1987; Siegel, 1983).

On the basis of these conditioning principles, Bootzin has formulated one of the most popular conceptual models of human insomnia—the stimulus control paradigm (Bootzin, 1972; Bootzin & Nicassio, 1978). For good sleepers, various stimuli such as the bed, bedroom, or bedtime have acquired discriminative control, in that they are potent cues associated with drowsiness and sleep onset. Conversely, for poor sleepers these same stimuli are often associated with frustration, arousal, and sleeplessness. According to this paradigm, when situational (bed/bedroom) and temporal (bedtime) stimuli are repeatedly paired with sleep-incompatible activities (overt or covert in nature), these stimuli gradually lose their discriminative properties previously associated with sleep. For example, when an individual routinely engages in nonsleeping activities (reading, watching TV, listening to the radio) in the bedroom, these cues are no longer associated with sleep. Likewise, a person who uses bedtime to solve problems, to rehash events of the day, or simply to worry about the inability to sleep eventually associates this particular time with frustration and sleeplessness. These various stimuli then lead to a conditioned arousal, which may manifest itself in terms of physiological, cognitive, or emotional activation, all of which are sleep-incompatible.

Only two investigations have attempted to empirically validate this conceptualization (Haynes, Adams, West, Kamens, & Safranek, 1982; Kazarian, Howe, & Csapo, 1979). In one study (Haynes et al., 1982), self-defined insomniacs did not report a higher rate of overt sleep-incompatible behaviors than good sleepers, nor was there a significant relationship between the frequency of these behaviors and subjective sleep latency. In contrast, Kazarian et al. (1979) found that insomniacs engaged more often in both overt (reading, eating, listening to the radio) and covert (negative thoughts at bedtime) activities; however, these authors also pointed out that not all behaviors reported to occur in the bedroom surroundings (e.g., pleasant conversation, sex) were sleep-incompatible. Additional research, using concurrent rather than retrospective measures of these activities and clinical rather than analogue populations, is needed to further validate this paradigm. Nevertheless, this model has enjoyed great popularity among clinicians and has led to one of the most effective treatment methods for insomnia— stimulus control therapy.

## An Integrative Model of Insomnia

The various paradigms reviewed thus far are theoretically sound, and each of them provides a clinical rationale lending itself to a different treatment modality. There is, however, no single paradigm that can account for the various insomnia subtypes. Insomnia is a multidimensional problem, not a unitary phenomenon, and most of the etiological mechanisms reviewed above are complementary rather than mutually exclusive. To facilitate a better understanding of this disorder and to enable clinicians to design more effective interventions, a conceptual framework integrating several lines of converging evidence is outlined here. In the first section of this chapter, an overview of the natural history of insomnia has been discussed. To conclude the chapter, I present a microanalytic view of insomnia (see Figure 4.2) that emphasizes the interactions between and among organismic, temporal, and environmental variables. The stimulus–organism–response–consequence model derived from social learning theory provides a useful conceptual framework (see Haynes & O'Brien, 1990) for examining the interrelationships among these variables.

1. Hyperarousal is the central mediating feature of insomnia. Because arousal regulates the balance between sleep and wakefulness, an excessive level of arousal is incompatible with sleep. This can be manifested in several channels: verbal (cognitive–affective), motoric (behavioral), and physiological (central and autonomic nervous systems). The literature on anxiety disorders indicates that these response systems are rarely synchronized with one another, in that excessive cognitive activation (intrusive thoughts) may or may not be paralleled by autonomic hyperactivity (increased heart rate, temperature, muscle tension). Even within a given response system (physiological), correlations among different measures (e.g., heart rate, skin conductance) are fairly modest, though affective and cognitive variables may be more strongly

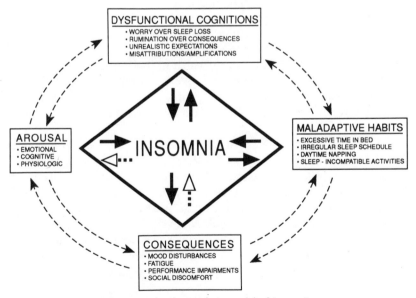

**FIGURE 4.2.** A microanalytic model of insomnia.

interrelated within the verbal domain. Manifestations of arousal may predominate in one channel for a given insomniac, whereas another may express it in a completely different modality. Thus, the first assumption is that hyperarousal (i.e., emotional, cognitive, physiological) is the common pathway to insomnia. It has primarily a causal influence on sleep disturbances, though it may also be exacerbated by sleeplessness.

2. A variety of stimulus conditions can elevate arousal above a critical threshold, such that it interrupts the natural sequence of relaxation, drowsiness, and sleep onset. For example, after several poor nights' sleep, a person may come to associate certain temporal (bedtime routines) and contextual (bedroom surroundings) stimuli with apprehensions, worries, and fear of being unable to sleep. The speed with which this conditioning process takes place varies across people; perhaps those individuals who are already more prone to insomnia may also be more susceptible to conditioning. Because nighttime sleep is also dependent on daytime activities, the stimulus conditions leading to insomnia may involve aversive events occurring during the day. Insomniacs may be more reactive and may take longer to recover from what most people would consider daily routine hassles. As such, a variety of problematic situations or interpersonal conflicts encountered during the day may serve as activating events leading to sleeplessness at night. If insomniacs internalize psychological conflicts, they may remain "worked up" even at bedtime. Negative daytime events may then fuel arousal at bedtime and strengthen the underlying conditioning process.

3. The most typical responses to sleeplessness include worries over sleep loss, ruminations about the daytime residual effects, muscle tension, and a general bodily restlessness. Along with these reactions, there is a universal tendency to try harder to go to sleep, which in itself enhances performance anxiety. Excessive arousal causes perceptual distortions of elapsed time, which further accentuate subjective sleep difficulties and distress. Eventually, the sleep drive becomes compelling enough that it overrides all these competing factors.

4. The next-day consequences involve fatigue, mood disturbances (irritability), social discomfort, and performance impairments. These perceived sequelae, whether accurate or amplified, only remind an individual of how miserable sleep was on the preceding night and trigger further dysfunctional cognitions about oneself and about sleep. Over time, a sense of learned helplessness becomes engrained, and chronic insomniacs come to believe that their insomnia is uncontrollable, unpredictable, and solely attributable to external causes. Inevitably, these negative self-statements set the individuals up for a chain reaction of emotional upset, more cognitive arousal, and further sleep disturbances.

5. In order to cope with insomnia, people may develop maladaptive sleep habits (e.g., excessive time spent in bed, irregular sleep–wake schedules,

and daytime napping). Although these coping strategies may temporarily minimize sleep loss, over the long run they interfere with the synchronizing effect of a regular and constrained sleep–wake rhythm. Transient use of hypnotic medications may also improve sleep, but with long-term use it eventually becomes part of the problem. Cognitive distortions (e.g., faulty beliefs about sleep-promoting practices, unrealistic expectations, mis-attributions of the causes of insomnia, and amplifications of its consequences) produce emotional distress and aggravate the insomnia problem further.

As I have noted throughout this book, chronic insomnia does not develop overnight. It is almost always preceded by situational insomnia that was brought on by stressful life events, but that failed to improve even after the stressors were removed. As such, it can evolve in a gradual fashion, so that the individual becomes progressively more absorbed by the sleep problem and by its presumed impact on daytime functioning. Appraisal of the initial sleep difficulty is a determining factor of whether it will be a transient problem or develop into full-fledged chronic insomnia. For instance, the individual who experiences several nights of poor sleep, but goes on with his or her usual routine without worrying about it, is unlikely to develop persistent insomnia. Conversely, a person who after a few nights of disturbed sleep becomes overly concerned with sleeplessness and its negative consequences on daytime functioning is likely to enter a vicious cycle of insomnia, emotional and cognitive arousal, and further sleep disturbances. Excessive rumination about sleeplessness quickly becomes the center of the person's preoccupations. Performance impairment or mood disturbances during the day tend to be exclusively attributed to poor sleep. Apprehension builds up in the evening, and as bedtime approaches, fearfulness of being unable to sleep becomes magnified. Following a poor night's sleep, not only does the individual worry about the previous night, but he or she already anticipates the next one with apprehension. Hence, insomnia becomes a self-fulfilling prophecy.

As can be seen from this model, the consequences of sleeplessness often become the causes and vice versa. There is a bidirectional influence among these controlling variables, and it becomes almost impossible to disentangle their causal relationships (Haynes & O'Brien, 1990). For all practical purposes, it may not be essential to do so, as both factors are directly addressed in treatment. This conceptual framework has several implications for the management of chronic insomnia. First, learned behavioral and cognitive responses play a major contributory role in maintaining insomnia. Treatment should thus focus not so much on uncovering the precipitating events as on altering its perpetuating conditions. The primary targets for intervention are the maladaptive sleep habits and dysfunctional sleep cognitions. Second, attempts at teaching insomniacs to directly control the sleep process may backfire and exacerbate performance anxiety. It is preferable to train them in controlling the temporal, contextual, behavioral, and cognitive factors that facilitate sleep. After the clinician has ensured that the timing of sleep is set according to circadian principles (temporal) in an environment that is conducive to sleep (contextual), treatment must focus on modifying maladaptive sleep habits (behavioral) and dysfunctional cognitions (affective–cognitive).

# 5

## Assessment of the Insomnia Patient

The effective management of insomnia requires a comprehensive evaluation of its nature, severity, and natural history, and a detailed functional analysis of its contributing factors. Although this is true of any clinical problem, a common mistake is to view insomnia as a simple symptomatic disorder. Consequently, treatment is often initiated prematurely without the benefit of an adequate evaluation. Because insomnia is associated with multiple causal factors, a detailed investigation of its controlling variables is essential prior to initiating treatment. This chapter reviews the typical assessment procedures used in our clinic. Measures designed primarily for research purposes are summarized, and their usefulness for clinical practice is discussed.

A multitrait–multimethod approach, involving several assessment devices tapping various facets of insomnia, is ideal for obtaining the most thorough evaluation. The measures administered include preliminary screening questionnaires and symptom checklists, a clinical interview, sleep diary monitoring, and psychological screening. Various ancillary measures, nocturnal polysomnography, and behavioral assessment devices may also be employed at the examiner's discretion.

After the initial contact with a prospective patient, several paper-and-pencil measures are mailed along with sleep diaries to be completed prior to the initial interview. Basic demographic data and information on presenting sleep symptomatology can thus be obtained in a systematic and economical fashion. By reviewing this preliminary information before the interview, the clinician can get some understanding of the patient's sleep difficulties and can identify specific areas in need of further evaluation.

### The Clinical Interview

To clarify and validate the initial information obtained from the screening questionnaires, a detailed review of the sleep problem is conducted with the patient during the clinical interview. The clinician's role is to obtain a comprehensive evaluation of the sleep problem and of potential contributing factors in a relatively short period of time. A directive style focusing on sleep relevant materials is most effective. My colleagues and I have designed over the past several years the Insomnia Interview Schedule (Appendix A), which has proved a useful instrument for eliciting in a cost-effective manner information clinically relevant to the assessment and diagnosis of insomnia. This interview is conducted in a semistructured format and takes 1 to 1.5 hours to administer. It is designed to obtain a sleep history; to screen for other sleep disorders; and to gauge the relative contribution of psychological, behavioral, environmental, and medical factors. It also provides guidelines for conducting a functional analysis investigating antecedents, consequences, secondary gains, precipitating factors, and perpetuating factors. This interview schedule is intended for use primarily with individuals presenting with a complaint of insomnia. The focus of the evaluation and the type of inquiries would vary substantially for those with disorders of excessive sleepiness or with features of parasomnias. The most important components of insomnia assessment are a detailed history and a careful functional analysis of its controlling variables (Bootzin & Engle-Friedman, 1981; Spielman, 1986). Accordingly, several facets of the insomnia problem are targeted during the assessment interview.

## The Sleep History

### NATURE OF THE COMPLAINT

The nature of the complaint is the first element considered: problems with falling asleep, trouble staying asleep, early-morning awakening, light sleep, nonrestorative or unrefreshing sleep, or impairments of daytime functioning. These descriptors reflect on the subjective and heterogeneous nature of insomnia. Difficulty in initiating and difficulty in maintaining sleep are not exclusive of each other; a person may present with sleep-onset, sleep-maintenance, or mixed sleep-onset and sleep-maintenance insomnia. Trouble sustaining sleep may involve brief but frequent awakenings, infrequent but prolonged awakenings, or early-morning awakening with inability to return to sleep. It is also necessary to distinguish between complaints of insomnia and hypersomnia. Although these can coexist, the latter usually reflects a different sleep pathology (e.g., sleep apnea, narcolepsy). Finally, the chief complaint should be distinguished from its presumed consequences. Fatigue, irritability, and decreased performance efficiency are often blamed on poor sleep, and these factors often motivate a person to seek treatment. The nature of the initial complaint should guide the clinician for the remainder of the interview, as each presenting symptom is typically associated with different physical and psychological correlates.

Although mixed features of anxiety and depression are common among insomniacs, the former is more frequently associated with trouble falling asleep, whereas the latter is more common in those with difficulties in sustaining sleep. Sleep apnea or periodic limb movements may lead to a complaint of sleep-maintenance insomnia, though they are more often linked with excessive daytime sleepiness. Some medical problems (e.g., esophageal reflux) are more likely to cause sleep-maintenance than sleep-onset problems. Some patients report daytime sleepiness as their initial problem, but further inquiry often reveals that fatigue instead of true sleepiness is the presenting problem. In fact, psychophysiological insomniacs tend to be hyperaroused and more alert than good sleepers during the day as well as at night (Stepanski et al., 1988; Sugerman et al., 1985).

SLEEP–WAKE SCHEDULE

The patient's typical sleep–wake schedule is examined next. The usual "sleep window" (initial bedtime and final arising time) is determined first, so as to obtain an estimate of the typical amount of time spent in bed. It also clarifies the timing of sleep and wakefulness throughout the 24-hour day. Bedtime and time of retiring may differ, as some people read in bed for variable durations before turning out the lights. Likewise, the last time of awakening is distinguished from the actual arising time. Premature awakenings that are spontaneous should be differentiated from scheduled ones or those triggered by environmental factors (e.g., a hot room, a crying baby, a barking dog). In addition, the duration of the previous sleep period should be considered, instead of relying exclusively on the actual clock time of the last awakening. For example, waking up at 4:00 A.M. has different diagnostic implications, depending on whether bedtime was 9:00 or 11:00 P.M.

The frequency and duration of daytime naps, both intentional and unintentional ones, should be explored. Even brief periods of dozing off should be examined, as these may also interfere with nighttime sleep. Insomniacs often report that regardless of how hard they try, they can never nap. Others deny napping but admit to nodding off when they do not intend to (e.g., while reading or watching TV). These statements illustrate the type of performance anxiety inhibiting sleep onset in chronic insomnia sufferers.

Variability in sleep schedules, either from night to night or from weekdays to weekends, should be explored to distinguish the primary insomnias from those attributable to sleep–wake schedule disorders. Individuals operating on irregular or unconventional sleep schedules (e.g., night and rotating shift workers) may present with a chief complaint of insomnia. The underlying disorder in such cases, however, is usually a sleep–wake schedule problem resulting from desynchronization of internal circadian rhythms, and treatment recommendations may vary accordingly.

## INSOMNIA SEVERITY

Several indices can be used to gauge the severity of insomnia. Global estimates of sleep-onset latency, number and duration of awakenings, and total sleep time provide a useful subjective index of insomnia intensity. The temporal distribution of night wakings should be clarified, as well as whether they are spontaneous, scheduled (i.e., with an alarm clock), or triggered by other factors (e.g., pain, nocturia, a crying baby). Because there is so much night to night variability in their sleep patterns, most insomniacs have difficulties in estimating these parameters. In eliciting this information, the clinician should provide a specific time frame (e.g., the past month) on which they can base their estimates of a typical night's sleep. It should be clarified whether important changes in the sleep pattern have occurred during this period; such changes may occur when a person has just started or has recently stopped taking hypnotic medications.

The patient's retrospective figures are only rough estimates and should not be taken at face value. Not unlike a patient's sleep diary data as compared with EEG data, the patient's retrospective estimates of sleep parameters can grossly amplify the problem's severity. As a minimum, these estimates must always be supplemented with daily sleep diary monitoring. At this evaluative stage, however, only preliminary data are needed, and the patient's subjective perception should not be challenged.

The number of nights per week a person experiences disturbed sleep is another good index of insomnia severity. Whether a patient has trouble sleeping night after night or one or two nights per week provides additional clues about the nature and intensity of the problem. It is unusual for insomniacs, even for those with chronic and severe problems, to experience trouble sleeping every single night. When it does occur nightly, the clinician may be more suspicious of an underlying psychological or medical basis for the insomnia.

## DAYTIME SEQUELAE OF INSOMNIA

Assessing the impact of disturbed sleep on daytime functioning and on the quality of life is important for gauging the clinical significance of insomnia. Is decreased sleep duration strictly a clinical phenomenon, or is it such a significant problem that it has become the central concern of a patient's life? Sleeplessness is not necessarily pathological. Individuals with decreased sleep duration without any concomitant daytime consequences may simply be natural short sleepers falling at the end of a normal continuum; they should not be considered insomniacs. The sequelae most commonly attributed to poor sleep include daytime mood disturbances (e.g., irritability), fatigue, social discomfort, and impairment of cognitive and behavioral performance

(Zammit, 1988). These presumed consequences are not necessarily corroborated by objective measurement. However, it is important to examine the patient's subjective perception of how his or her life is affected by chronic insomnia. These clinical issues will be directly addressed in the cognitive therapy module.


THE NATURAL HISTORY OF INSOMNIA

The clinical interview continues with a review of the natural history of insomnia. Specific issues of inquiry include the onset, duration, and time course. The duration is perhaps the most important factor in distinguishing between situational (days or weeks) and chronic (months or years) insomnia. Although many patients claim to have experienced sleep difficulty as long as they can remember, the clinician needs to work backward through specific phases of the life cycle to determine whether the onset occurred in childhood, adolescence, young adulthood, middle age, or late life. Early versus late onset may have different implications for treatment outcome, with childhood onset presenting a poorer prognosis (Edinger et al., 1988; Lacks & Powlishta, 1989). Likewise, a sudden as opposed to a gradual onset may have more readily identifiable precipitating events, and treatment may vary accordingly. The most common instigating factors are stressful life events such as family-, health-, and work-related difficulties (Healy et al., 1981). With early-onset insomnia, possible physical or sexual abuse during childhood should be investigated. The onset of insomnia during menopause may be linked to hormonal changes occuring during this life cycle (Ballinger, 1976).

     The time course of insomnia and its intensity should be scrutinized, as these may provide additional etiological clues. Does sleep pattern fluctuate weekly, monthly, or seasonally, or is it persistent without remission periods? Recurring but episodic insomnia may be indicative of concomitant medical or psychological problems. Sleep disruptions may be more severe during the spring season in those whose insomnia is secondary to allergies. Patients with seasonal affective disorder may also present with periodic variations in their sleep patterns. Bipolar patients are insomniac during the manic phase and hypersomniac during the depressive cycle. College students with sleep disturbances often experience temporary relief during vacation breaks. Psychophysiological insomniacs, however, generally report having suffered persistent sleep difficulties with few if any remission periods. The only exception may be when they go away from home and experience a temporary and surprising relief, though many refuse to leave home, fearing that their sleep problem will become even worse in a surrounding to which they are not accustomed.

## ENVIRONMENTAL FACTORS

Environmental factors assume a salient role in precipitating and perpetuating sleep disturbances. Light, noise, room temperature, and mattress comfort are obvious factors that may interfere with normal sleep and should not be overlooked. Their potential influence is especially noteworthy for hospitalized patients or nursing home residents, who often share bedrooms and have to adjust to others' sleep environment preferences. The clinician should systematically evaluate the impact of the physical environment on sleep disruptions.

## MEDICATION USE

Taking a complete drug history is essential in the evaluation of insomnia, as many different drugs can alter sleep. Long-term use of sedative–hypnotics is a major perpetuating factor of insomnia. Other psychotropic medications and those prescribed for physical illnesses (e.g., beta-blockers, bronchodilators, steroids), as well as over-the-counter sleep aids, should be identified. The dosage, frequency, duration of usage, and the patient's response to the drugs should be evaluated. Long-acting benzodiazepines can have daytime residual effects impairing alertness and performance. These deficits are often mistakenly attributed to disturbed sleep, whereas they may simply represent residual effects from the previous night's drug use. Use of alcohol and psychoactive drugs (e.g., marijuana, cocaine, amphetamines) should be examined, as well as prior history of abuse and/or treatment for chemical dependency. A table listing the most common drugs affecting sleep is provided in Chapter 2.

In gathering this information, the clinician should examine the patient's attitudes toward drugs. Although a large number of patients meet diagnostic criteria for drug-dependent insomnia, many of them have negative attitudes toward drug-taking, but feel trapped in this psychological dependency. Conversely, a few individuals are essentially seeking drug treatment or renewal of a prescription that a primary care physician refuses to refill. The clinician needs to be alert to these cases. It is essential to examine the patient's acceptance of a nondrug intervention and to explore the level of intended compliance with such a treatment regimen (Morin, Gaulier, Barry, & Kowatch, 1992).

## DIETARY, SMOKING, AND EXERCISE HABITS

Caffeine and nicotine are both central nervous system stimulants, and as such are sleep-disrupting substances. Information on their intake (particularly in the evening) should be obtained and, when necessary, supplemented by more systematic monitoring on the daily sleep diary. The types and quantity of food and liquid consumed near bedtime should be assessed to determine their potential etiological contribution. Excessive liquid intake can lead to nocturia, especially in older people with reduced bladder capacity. The frequency and timing of aerobic exercise also needs to be evaluated, as strenuous exercise performed too close to bedtime may be overstimulating and delay sleep onset.

## SCREENING FOR OTHER SLEEP DISORDERS

A review of the most commmon symptoms of other sleep pathology is essential to reach a preliminary differential diagnosis between primary insomnia and insomnia secondary to other sleep disorders. This task is best accomplished with the bed partner, because the patient is usually unaware of these occult symptoms occuring only during sleep. Section 8 of the Insomnia Interview Schedule lists the most common symptoms associated with restless-legs syndrome, periodic limb movements, sleep apnea, narcolepsy, gastroesophageal reflux, and some of the parasomnias. Their diagnostic features are also described in Chapter 3. Most of these disorders, however, can only be diagnosed or definitely ruled out by nocturnal polysomnography.

## MEDICAL HISTORY

A medical history is important to clarify the role of factors such as pain, anemia, and hyperthyroidism. The medical history should include at a minimum a list of drugs currently used, active physical illness, prior surgery, and hospitalizations. We do not require younger patients who are apparently healthy to undergo a physical examination prior to treatment. However, in older people without a recent physical exam, and in patients of any age with evidence of a contributing medical factor or symptoms of sleep apnea (e.g., snoring, obesity, daytime sleepiness), a complete physical examination is obtained.

Even when a medical problem is present, it does not necessarily mean that the insomnia is secondary in nature. Despite the widespread coexistence of sleep and medical disorders, learned behavioral factors almost always play a major role in long-term insomnia. Separate therapeutic attention may be required, whether or not it is associated with a physical problem. In any case, the level of interference with sleep caused by medical problems should be gauged. For example, chronic pain often leads to sleep disturbances, and the interaction of these two conditions as well as their fluctuation over time should be evaluated (Morin & Gramling, 1990).

By now the clinician has a general understanding of the nature, perceived severity, and natural history of the sleep problem. The potential role of medical, environmental, and pharmacological factors has been examined. The next step involves a much more detailed and refined analysis of the insomnia problem.

## A Functional Analysis

Conducting a comprehensive functional analysis of antecedents, consequences, and other controlling variables is essential to understanding insomnia. This involves investigating the situational, organismic, and temporal variables that either alleviate or exacerbate sleep difficulties (Bootzin & Engle-Friedman, 1981; Spielman, 1986). The functional analysis enables the clinician to identify the perpetuating factors and to tailor a rational intervention adapted to these difficulties (Haynes & O'Brien, 1990).

Careful inquiry about the patient's prebedtime routines, sleep-incompatible activities, secondary gains, and typical responses to sleeplessnes is a critical component of the evaluation process. For example, is bedtime a prime time for problem solving with a spouse, for rehashing events of the day at work, or for planning tomorrow's schedule? Does the patient engage in sleep-interfering activities in the bedroom, such as watching TV, listening to the radio, or talking on the telephone? Or does he or she read in bed during the day or at bedtime? Is there an office set up in the bedroom with a desk for doing paperwork and paying the bills? Sleep-incompatible activities can either be cognitive (covert) or behavioral (overt) in nature. Therefore, inquiry about specific self-statements occurring in regard to bed-related stimuli is as important as inquiry about overt sleep-incompatible behaviors. Is the patient apprehensive about bedtime? How is this processed cognitively? What does the patient do or say to himself or herself when unable to fall asleep or return to sleep in the middle of the night? Inadequate stimulus control is one of the main etiological paradigms for insomnia (Bootzin & Nicassio, 1978; Bootzin, Epstein, & Wood, 1991). When sleep-incompatible behaviors are repeatedly performed at or near bedtime and in the bedroom surroundings, temporal (bedtime) and environmental (bed/bedroom) stimuli may come to lose their discriminative properties previously associated with sleep. A careful inquiry about these practices will help identify perpetuating conditions. It may also enhance the patient's understanding of the rationale and acceptability of stimulus control therapy, which is directly derived from this conceptual model.

Secondary gains play a greater role in maintaining sleep disturbances than is generally assumed. Although insomniacs are usually ashamed of their lack of control over sleep and do not publicize these difficulties, potential secondary gains should be explored. This is best accomplished by evaluating how a patient's life is affected by sleep disturbances. It is not unusual for poor sleepers to restrict family involvement, social interactions, and general activity level, or to make these contingent upon the quality and duration of the previous night's sleep. Time off from work, sympathy from family members or coworkers, and avoidance of family or social obligations may contribute to maintaining sleep disturbances. Sleeping in a different bedroom than a spouse may be a more acceptable manner of avoiding intimacy, even though the main reason advanced may be that the patient does not want to disturb the bedmate or that the bedmate snores too loudly. Finally, the anxiolytic properties of most benzodiazepines may prove a powerful secondary reinforcer and contribute to continuing drug dependency.

The unpredictability of sleep is one of the core features of psychophysiological insomnia. Typically, a good night's sleep is interspersed with several poor ones. After two or three nights of disturbed sleep, the individual is usually so exhausted that sleep comes more easily. Another struggle ensues on the following night, and the cycle goes on and on. With nightly fluctuations in sleep patterns, it is easier to conduct a functional analysis of the alleviating and exacerbating factors. For some people, going away on vacation may provide temporary insomnia relief, since the situational cues leading to poor sleep at home are no longer present in a different surrounding. For others, the anticipatory anxiety associated with sleeping in a strange environment unavoidably leads to even more disrupted sleep when they are away from home. Differences in sleep quality between weekdays and weekends can shed light on the role played by occupational stress.

Insomnia should never be evaluated strictly as a nighttime problem. What poor sleepers think, do, and feel during the day can clearly have an impact on nighttime sleep (Marchini et al., 1983). Daytime cognitions, behaviors, and affect should be examined. Excessive worry over sleep loss and daytime deficits, or apprehension about the upcoming night's sleep, can set the stage for another sleepless night. In patients with anxiety features, sleep is often worse on weeknights because of apprehension about performance deficits at work. On weekends, there is less worry about these daytime deficits, and sleep is improved. "Sunday night insomnia" may stem from the anticipatory anxiety of returning to work or from sleep accumulation over the weekend. This phenomenon is common even in good sleepers, who catch up on weekends and are just not sleepy by their usual bedtime on Sunday nights.

Taking a comprehensive sleep history and conducting a careful behavioral analysis are the two most important components of insomnia assessment. Because there are numerous factors leading to the complaint of insomnia, this evaluation should be done in a systematic fashion. Support and empathy is important, but the clinician should also take a directive and problem-oriented approach.

## Sleep Diary Monitoring

Self-monitoring of various target behaviors has proved an invaluable assessment tool for many clinical dysfunctions. Similarly, the use of sleep diary monitoring is one of the key elements in the evaluation of insomnia (Bootzin & Engle-Friedman, 1981; Spielman, 1986). A typical sleep diary requires daily recording of the following parameters: bedtime, arising time, sleep-onset latency, number and duration of awakenings, time of last awakening, naps, medication intake, and some indices of sleep quality. These variables are coded as follows: Sleep-onset latency (abbreviated as SOL in the diary; see Appendices F and G) is defined as the time from initial lights-out to sleep onset; wake after sleep onset (WASO) refers to the amount of time awake from the initial sleep onset to the last awakening; early-morning awakening (EMA) is the time awake from the last awakening until final arising time; total wake time (TWT) is the summation of SOL + WASO + EMA. The next step consists of calculating the "sleep window," which is defined as the total time elapsed from initial time in bed to final time out of bed. This variable is typically referred to as time in bed (TIB); however, it should also include the time patients may have spent out of bed during this period, either by choice or because they were required to do so during treatment. Total sleep time (TST) is obtained by subtracting TWT from TIB. Finally, a sleep efficiency ratio (SE) is obtained by dividing TST by TIB (the "sleep window") and multiplying by 100. After these variables are coded for each night, a weekly mean is computed.

The diary provided in Appendix F has proved extremely useful for both clinical and research purposes. It is simple to use, and its design gives a quick pictorial display of a patient's sleep patterns for an entire week. The clinician can at a glance gain an understanding of the nature, frequency, and intensity of insomnia; of nightly variations in sleep schedules; and of some common perpetuating factors (e.g., daytime naps, medication intake). It may be simplified or altered depending on a patient's specific needs. At the very least, it should include estimates of time in bed, sleep time, and wake time, so that a global sleep efficiency ratio can be calculated. Patients are required to complete at least 2 weeks of sleep logs before starting treatment and throughout the intervention thereafter. A weekly summary data sheet (Appendix G) is available to enable clinician and patient to review progress at each therapy session. Instructions for completing the diary are provided, along with an example printed directly on the diary. Some patients may require training in completing this form. The clinician should make sure to review the diary at each visit and to provide corrective feedback when needed; this will underscore the importance placed on this assessment device. Because of an underlying obsessive cognitive style, some insomniacs are fairly concerned about providing the most accurate data. Despite the importance of keeping accurate daily records, clock watching should be discouraged.

Maintaining a daily sleep diary serves several purposes. First, it helps establish a baseline of the initial severity of the sleep problem. Patients may realize after a few days of self-monitoring that they get more sleep than they initially thought. Enhanced awareness may decrease the patients' anxiety over sleep loss, and consequently may alleviate the subjective complaints. It also provides a better understanding of how sleep patterns change over time and can pinpoint situational and temporal factors contributing to these variations. The sleep diary is also an excellent tool for monitoring progress over the course of treatment. It is not unusual for some patients to lose track of how disturbed their sleep was at baseline, and consequently to fail to recognize improvements. By monitoring progress and providing weekly feedback, the diary will enhance such patients' awareness that progress has indeed been made. Finally, compliance with keeping the diary provides a test of expected compliance with the intervention.

The main drawbacks of sleep diary monitoring have to do with convergent validity, reactivity, and compliance. There are variations among subjective, behavioral, and physiological sleep measures. For example, insomniacs have a tendency to overestimate sleep-onset latency and underestimate sleep duration in comparison to EEG measurement (Carskadon et al., 1976; Coates et al., 1982; Frankel et al., 1976). However, daily morning estimates of specific sleep parameters (sleep-onset latency or wake after sleep onset) yield a reliable and valid relative index of insomnia, even though they do not reflect absolute values obtained from polysomnography (Coates et al., 1982). These daily estimates are also less subject to exaggeration than is a single, global, and retrospective measure; as such, they represent a more acceptable compromise. The problem of reactivity can be attenuated by extending baseline monitoring for at least 2 weeks, which is the standard in current outcome research (Lacks & Morin, 1992). Compliance with daily monitoring is usually not a major problem. However, some researchers require their subjects to mail or call in their diary data on a daily basis (Friedman, Bliwise, Yesavage, & Salom, 1991; Lacks, Bertelson, Gans, & Kunkel, 1983; Spielman, Saskin, & Thorpy, 1987). In clinical practice, this requirement may not be practical or readily accepted by patients.

In summary, although self-report of sleep variables is prone to the same problems of validity, reliability, and reactivity that affect self-monitoring in general, daily sleep diary monitoring is still the most practical, most economical, and the most widely used method for assessing insomnia (Bootzin & Engle-Friedman, 1981). Despite some limitations, the low cost of sleep diaries allows for prospectively tracking sleep patterns over extensive periods of time, thereby yielding a more representative sample of a person's sleep than one or two nights of polysomnography can do. This is particularly important in light of the extensive night-to-night variability in sleep patterns of chronic insomniacs (Espie, Lindsay, Brooks, Hood, & Turvey, 1989).

## Psychological Screening

A psychological screening evaluation is routinely performed on all patients in our clinic. It involves obtaining a history of current and past psychiatric treatment and hospitalization, reviewing symptoms for major psychopathology, and administering several psychological inventories. A detailed inquiry of recent life experiences is helpful to evaluate the role of stressful events (e.g., family or marital conflicts, occupational stress, birth of a child, financial strains) in the development of sleep disturbances. In addition, all patients are administered the following instruments: the Brief Symptom Inventory (Derogatis & Melisaratos, 1983); the Beck Depression Inventory (Beck, Ward, Mendelson, Mock, & Erbaugh, 1961); the State–Trait Anxiety Inventory (Spielberger, Gorsuch, & Lushene, 1970) or the Beck Anxiety Inventory (Beck, Epstein, Brown, & Steer, 1988); and the Profile of Mood States (McNair, Lorr, & Droppleman, 1971).

This psychological screening assessment should be an integral part of the evaluation process for several reasons. First, there is a high prevalence of psychopathology among insomniacs. When disturbed sleep is strictly a symptom of more severe psychopathology, treatment should be directed at the underlying psychiatric condition. To this end, the Brief Symptom Inventory provides useful data about global psychological distress and can guide the clinician in deciding whether a more detailed evaluation is needed to confirm or rule out major psychopathology. Second, although most insomnia sufferers may not meet criteria for a major depressive disorder or a generalized anxiety disorder, the majority present with mixed features of depression and/or anxiety. The intensity of these clinical features can easily be evaluated with the Beck inventories and the State–Trait Anxiety Inventory. Third, mood disturbances are common sequelae attributed to poor sleep. The Profile of Mood States is an excellent instrument to evaluate such mood disturbances and to track their temporal fluctuations associated with changes in sleep patterns during the course of treatment.

Although a more complete evaluation can be performed when there is evidence of severe psychopathology, this screening assessment is sufficient for most insomnia patients. Time is best invested in administering instruments more directly linked to the sleep problem and more likely to yield data clinically relevant to treatment planning and outcome assessment.

## Ancillary Measures

The Sleep Impairment Index (Appendix B) is a 7-item measure that yields a quantitative index of sleep impairment. The patient provides ratings (on a 5-point scale) of the severity, degree of interference with daily functioning, noticeability of impairment attributed to the sleep problem, level of distress caused by the sleep problem, and satisfaction with current sleep patterns. These subjective ratings provide valuable information on the patient's perception of his or her sleep problem. A parallel version of this scale is also completed by the clinician and by a significant other (e.g., spouse, roommate) to provide collateral validation of treatment outcome. Significant correlations between these collateral ratings and diary data have been obtained (Morin & Azrin, 1985).

The Beliefs and Attitudes about Sleep Scale (Appendix C) is a 30-item questionnaire designed to tap sleep-related cognitions. Five theoretical factors are covered: misconceptions about the causes of insomnia; misattributions or amplification of its consequences; unrealistic expectations; control and predictability of sleep; and faulty beliefs about sleep-promoting practices. This instrument has proved extremely useful as a therapeutic tool for conducting cognitive therapy sessions. It helps to identify dysfunctional sleep-related cognitions and provides data on both treatment process and outcome. Patients complete this measure before their initial visit and at the conclusion of treatment. Hoelscher, Ware, and Bond (1993) have developed a similar instrument that measures more specifically the extent to which poor sleep is perceived to interfere with psychosocial and occupational functioning, mood, physical appearance, and so on.

Several additional paper-and-pencil measures have been designed to evaluate subjective dimensions of the sleep experience and theoretical constructs of insomnia. The first group of instruments is intended for use as a global and retrospective measure of sleep for various time intervals. The Pittsburgh Sleep Quality Index (Buysse, Reynolds, Monk, Berman, & Kupfer, 1989) is a 19-item instrument that assesses sleep quality over a 1-month time interval. Seven component scores (e.g., sleep quality, sleep-onset latency, duration, efficiency, disturbances, medication, and daytime dysfunction) are derived to yield a global score of sleep quality. This measure is not specific to insomnia, but it may yield useful information about sleep disturbances in general. The Sleep Behavior Self-Rating Scale (Kazarian et al., 1979) is a 24-item instrument assessing the frequency with which a person engages in sleep-incompatible practices in the bed/bedroom; as such, it is useful for gathering information about inadequate stimulus control. It discriminates well between poor and good sleepers when insomnia is defined as sleep-onset difficulties. The Arousal Predisposition Scale (Coren, 1988) is a 12-item self-report instrument designed to assess arousability as a relatively stable predisposition rather than a state strictly limited to the bedtime interval. It is a good predictor of sleep disturbances, but has not been validated with a clinical population. The Sleep Hygiene Awareness and Practice Scale (Lacks & Rotert, 1986) measures whether the subject believes various activities are beneficial, are disruptive, or have no effect on sleep, and whether several food, beverages, and nonprescription drugs contain caffeine. It also measures the extent to which sleep is disturbed by environmental factors and the frequency with which subjects engage in poor sleep hygiene practices. This instrument is useful to examine the role played by poor sleep hygiene in perpetuating insomnia. The factorial structure of several additional sleep questionnaires has been examined in an attempt to tailor treatment to specific insomnia-causing factors (Coyle & Watts, 1991; Espie, Brooks, & Lindsay, 1989).

A number of rating scales are also available for daily use with sleep diaries. The Pre-Sleep Arousal Scale (Nicassio et al., 1985) is a 16-item self-report questionnaire measuring cognitive (e.g., racing thoughts, worries) and somatic (e.g., heart racing, muscle tension) arousal states at bedtime. It yields two scores weighing the relative contribution of intrusive cognitions and physiological factors to sleep-onset difficulties. The Post-Sleep Inventory (Webb, Bonnet, & Blume, 1976) is a 29-item scale that measures subjective aspects of the previous sleep period. Upon morning awakening, each item is rated on a 13-point scale with bipolar anchor points arranged according to three time periods: presleep (asleep quickly vs. long time awake), during sleep (frequently awakened vs. uninterrupted sleep), and postsleep (woke up extremely tired vs. woke up as rested as possible). This inventory provides useful information about the subjective sleep experience.

All these measures are useful to the extent that they provide a better understanding of the subjective sleep experience and yield a quantitative index of insomnia. Although they may prove useful in a clinical context, very few have been used or shown to be sensitive to sleep pattern changes in outcome research. The time invested relative to the information gained should be considered prior to their routine use in clinical or research practice.

## Nocturnal Polysomnography

Nocturnal polysomnography is recognized as the "gold standard" for sleep measurement and provides the most comprehensive assessment of a sleep disorder. It is the only assessment modality yielding data about sleep stages. A polysomnographic evaluation involves all-night electrographic monitoring of sleep (EEG, EOG, EMG), respiration, EKG, oxygen desaturation, and leg movements. By definition, sleep precludes awareness of many abnormalities (breathing pauses, leg twitches, etc.); polysomnography is therefore essential for diagnosing and documenting the severity of such sleep disorders as sleep apnea, periodic limb movements, and narcolepsy. For insomnia sufferers, a laboratory evaluation is helpful in assessing the nature and severity of the sleep problem. It is also useful in determining the level of discrepancy between the subjective complaint and actual sleep disturbances. EEG monitoring also provides information about atypical polysomnographic features (e.g., alpha–delta sleep) that are otherwise undetectable. REM latency is considered a biological marker of major depression (Reynolds & Kupfer, 1987), and polysomnography may yield useful information for patients who deny depressive symptomatology and exclusively emphasize their sleeplessness. A single night of polysomnography can even be therapeutic in some cases: The data may show a patient that he or she is getting more sleep than actually perceived. A laboratory setting provides an ideal opportunity for observing behaviors (e.g., body movements) and for monitoring physiological variables (e.g., frontalis EMG) that can yield important clues on the role played by physiological arousal in sleep disturbances.

Despite the wealth of information provided by nocturnal polysomnography, its role in the assessment and differential diagnosis of chronic insomnia remains controversial. Although some researchers and clinicians claim that a face-to-face clinical interview is sufficient (A. Kales & Kales, 1984), others argue that laboratory findings can significantly alter initial diagnostic impressions (Edinger, Hoelscher, et al., 1989; Jacobs et al., 1988). The main point of contention is whether insomnia is primarily a symptom of underlying psychopathology or one associated with medically based disorders (e.g. sleep apnea, myoclonus). A recent study of 123 insomnia patients showed that in 49% of the cases sleep laboratory results added to, refuted, and/or failed to support the initial clinical impression (Jacobs et al., 1988). Although there is no doubt that polysomnographic evaluations can add to diagnostic precision, it is unclear whether the information gained is of sufficient clinical value to improve treatment recommendations and outcome. Furthermore, it is unlikely that one night of sleep laboratory evaluation will yield valid and reliable information on insomnia severity. The well known "first-night effect" (a worsening of sleep), or the more common "reverse first-night effect" in insomniacs, limits its clinical usefulness with these patients (Hauri & Olmstead, 1989; Trinder, 1988). Although sleep laboratory facilities are now available in most major medical centers, the high cost of polysomnographic evaluations also remains a deterrent to their routine use.

There are several clinical indications for polysomnography. Patients whose chief complaint is excessive daytime sleepiness should almost always be evaluated overnight, unless it is clear that this is attributable to insufficient sleep. For those whose presenting problem is insomnia, the nature of the complaint and presence of associated symptoms should guide this decision. Sleep-maintenance insomnia is more likely to be associated with apnea or periodic leg movements than is sleep-onset insomnia alone. Obesity, loud snoring, and morning headaches are common symptoms of sleep apnea and should be followed by a polysomnographic evaluation, regardless of whether the underlying complaint is insomnia or hypersomnia. Age is also an important factor, because the incidence of several sleep disorders (including apnea and periodic limb movements) increases across the life cycle. As such, an overnight evaluation is often indicated with older patients whose chief complaint is sleep-maintenance insomnia. Finally, if a patient is unresponsive to behavioral treatment, a polysomnographic evaluation may uncover a primary sleep disorder that was missed during the initial evaluation.

Technological advances have now made possible electrophysiological recording from the patient's home or any areas remote from the sleep lab. The data from ambulatory polysomnography are either simultaneously transmitted to the lab via telephone lines (Telediagnostic System) or are tape-recorded and stored on a cassette carried in a case by the patient (Oxford Medilog System) (McCall, Edinger, & Erwin, 1989; Sewitch & Kupfer, 1985). Naturalistic recording in the home environment is perhaps the greatest advantage of ambulatory monitoring. This may attenuate the "first-night effect" associated with sleep laboratory evaluation. Patients' acceptance of ambulatory monitoring is higher than that of laboratory monitoring (Hoelscher et al., 1987). There is no need to have a technician on duty all night, but the risk of artifacts and invalidation in some ambulatory studies is higher. The lack of behavioral observations from technicians also make some records more difficult to interpret.

In summary, before an overnight sleep evaluation is considered, a detailed sleep history should always be obtained, with information pertaining to the current sleep–wake schedule, physical problems, medication/substance use, and psychological status. This information combined with the sleep diary data will guide the clinician in making a preliminary diagnosis, in deciding whether an overnight sleep study is warranted, and in planning treatment.

## Behavioral Assessment Devices

Several innovative sleep assessment devices have been designed over the past several years to supplement the information obtained from sleep diaries and to curtail the cost associated with polysomnography. Although most of these devices are still being validated, some of them appear particularly promising because they are less expensive and can be more readily used on a nightly basis in the patient's home environment.

## Wrist Actigraph

The Wrist Actigraph is a small sensing device that is worn on the wrist and records motor activity (Hauri & Wisbey, 1992; Mullaney, Kripke, & Messin, 1980). This ambulatory monitoring system uses a microprocessor to record and store wrist activity along with actual clock time. Data are recovered and processed through microcomputer software. An algorithm is used for estimating sleep-onset latency, wake after sleep onset, total sleep time, and total recording time. A similar computer-assisted device monitoring both physical activity and heart rate has been used by other investigators for estimating sleep–wake parameters (Burnett et al., 1985). Global measures of sleep duration and total wake time as estimated from wrist actigraphy are highly correlated with polysomnographic recordings in good sleepers. However, mixed results have been obtained with insomniacs, especially when the absolute values of more discrete variables such as sleep-onset latency, wake after sleep onset, and number of awakenings are compared. These discrepancies are particularly pronounced with patients with low levels of behavioral activity while awake (e.g., depressed insomniacs). Although technical refinements are needed before this device can be routinely used, this type of microprocessor-based ambulatory recording is promising for outcome research.

## Sleep Assessment Device

The Sleep Assessment Device (Lichstein, Nickel, Hoelscher, & Kelley, 1982) works by generating a brief, soft tone at fixed intervals (usually every 10 minutes) throughout the night. After each tone, a tape recorder is activated for 10 seconds and records the patient's verbal response. Absence of a verbal response ("I'm awake") is interpreted as evidence of sleep. A night's sleep pattern can be reconstructed by reviewing the 10-second samples occurring at 10-minute intervals. A 1-minute tape is produced for each hour of recording. This device yields five sleep parameters: sleep-onset latency, number of awakenings, duration of awakenings, total sleep time, and sleep efficiency. Studies comparing these estimates against measures obtained from insomniac patients, bedmates, and polysomnographic evaluations have yielded excellent data supporting the validity and nonintrusiveness of this device (Espie, Lindsay, & Espie, 1989; Lichstein, Hoelscher, Eakin, & Nickel, 1983; Lichstein et al., 1982; Lichstein & Johnson, 1991). The device has also been used in two treatment studies (Espie, Lindsay, Brooks, et al., 1989; Hoelscher & Edinger, 1988). Because the Sleep Assessment Device uses time-sampling intervals, it tends to underestimate wakefulness slightly, compared to poly-somnography or subjective data.

A similar device, the Sleep Monitor, operates under the same principles (Birrell, 1983), but the patient responds to the auditory signal by depressing a button switch taped to the preferred hand. A built-in memory module records the pattern of signals and responses. The sleep monitor yields estimates of sleep-onset latencies almost identical to that of latency to stage 2 sleep and somewhat smaller than subjective estimates. This device has not been used as extensively as the Sleep Assessment Device.

## Switch-Activated Clock

The switch-activated clock consists of a remote hand-held switch connected to an electric or battery-operated clock (Franklin, 1981). A momentary switch connection is designed such that the clock runs only when pressure is applied to the switch lever. On retiring to bed, the patient activates the clock by holding the switch in his or her hand and depressing the lever with the thumb. Relaxation of thumb pressure upon falling asleep releases the switch lever and automatically stops the clock. By setting the clock at a pre-determined time, the patient can obtain an objective measure of sleep-onset latency. Validation of this device against polysomnographic measurement showed that the switch is released within 5–10 minutes of polysomnography-defined sleep onset, with the correspondence being closer to stage 2 than stage 1 sleep (Morin & Schoen, 1986; Viens, De Koninck, Van Den Bergen, Audet, & Christ, 1988). This device has been used in one treatment study as a means of validating subjective estimates of sleep latency and awakening duration (Morin & Azrin, 1988).

These behavioral assessment devices offer several advantages, even though they do not provide measures of sleep stages. First, they are more economical than nocturnal polysomnography. They can be self-administered and do not require trained technicians to conduct the assessment and score the sleep records. Second, most of these devices are unobtrusive and only minimally affect the sleep process being measured. Third, they have the marked advantage of allowing sleep monitoring in the natural environment. Since sleep patterns can fluctuate greatly from one setting to another, it is essential to obtain a representative picture of the patient's typical sleep pattern in the home environment. For both clinical and research purposes, these instruments have much to offer in terms of documenting insomnia severity and for tracking changes in sleep pattern over the course of treatment. Two of these devices (the Wrist Actigraph and the Sleep Assessment Device) are commercially available.

## Concluding Comment

A sleep evaluation should include at a minimum a detailed sleep history (including a medical history) and a functional analysis, 2 weeks' worth of sleep diary monitoring, and a psychological screening assessment. If polysomnography is unavailable, treatment can still be initiated as long as there is no evidence of an underlying disorder such as sleep apnea. The clinician should integrate the information and data obtained from the different sources of assessment to make a preliminary diagnosis and design an initial treatment plan. However, assessment is an ongoing and interactive process that does not end when treatment is initiated (Bootzin, 1985). On the basis of the clinician's improved understanding of the patient's problem and initial treatment response, further assessment may be needed as the intervention unfolds. This initial evaluation should determine whether a particular patient is a suitable candidate for the treatment protocol described in the following chapters. Patients whose chief complaint of insomnia is clearly secondary to major psychopathology should be treated first for the underlying psychiatric condition. In mixed cases presenting with insomnia and psychological disturbances or insomnia and pain as equally important features, clinical judgment should dictate the initial focus of treatment. Further guidelines on these issues are provided in the next two chapters.

# II

## TREATMENT

# 6

## Overview of Treatment Protocol

This chapter presents an overview of the insomnia treatment protocol. Its four therapy components, described in greater detail in the following chapters, are introduced. I also discuss the clinical features of typical patients suitable for this intervention, relative contraindications, and the customary setting for implementing treatment. The format, duration, and structure of treatment are described, and outlines for each therapy session are provided at the end of the chapter.

This intervention is psychological in nature, and its theoretical foundations are based on social learning principles. The predominant clinical emphasis is on cognitive-behavioral approaches. As such, dream analysis or psychodynamic interpretations of sleeplessness are not offered. The main focus is on current maladaptive behavioral patterns and dysfunctional cognitive styles that perpetuate sleep difficulties. The protocol involves three distinct modules featuring behavioral, cognitive, and educational components, each targeting a different facet of insomnia. An optional module on medication withdrawal is offered for individuals with habitual reliance on sleep aids. These four therapy components are implemented in a sequential fashion. The order of presentation is based on the more extensive empirical evidence supporting the behavioral procedures over the cognitive or educational ones; this sequence, however, can be altered according to the hierarchy of causal factors identified during the initial evaluation. Finally, this treatment protocol is not a fixed formula for all insomniacs. The clinical relevance of each therapy component should be based on an ongoing assessment process, and in many cases individually tailored procedures will need to be added.

### Behavioral Component

Insomnia sufferers frequently develop strategies for coping with their sleep difficulties and the presumed deleterious effects of these on daytime functioning. Spending excessive amounts of time in bed, sleeping late in the morning, and routine daytime napping often help people to cope with the short-term detrimental effects of insomnia. In the long run, however, these same coping strategies interfere with sleep and perpetuate insomnia problems. Accordingly, the behavioral therapy component involves a combination of stimulus control and sleep restriction procedures. These procedures, which represent the heart of the entire intervention, are designed to eliminate sleep-incompatible behaviors, to regulate the sleep–wake schedule, and to consolidate sleep over a shorter period of time spent in bed. Stimulus control and sleep restriction therapies were designed, respectively, by Richard Bootzin (Bootzin, 1972; Bootzin et al., 1991) and by Arthur Spielman (Glovinsky & Spielman, 1991; Spielman, Saskin, & Thorpy, 1987). There is extensive empirical evidence supporting their clinical effectiveness in the management of chronic insomnia (see Chapter 12).

## Cognitive Component

The cognitive therapy component consists essentially of cognitive restructuring techniques modeled after the work of Aaron Beck, Albert Ellis, and Donald Meichenbaum and adapted to insomnia problems. Contemporary theories of psychopathology are increasingly emphasizing the importance of maladaptive cognitions (e.g., faulty appraisal, unrealistic expectations, misattributions) in the etiology of various disorders. This perspective is particularly relevant to sleep disturbances, as many insomniacs entertain a variety of dysfunctional cognitions that often exacerbate what otherwise might have been transient sleep problems. The cognitive therapy component is directed at correcting unrealistic sleep expectations, revising false attributions about the causes of insomnia, and reappraising perceptions of its consequences on daytime functioning. A three-step process is typically followed for achieving these goals: (1) identifying patient-specific dysfunctional cognitions; (2) confronting and challenging their validity; and (3) replacing them with more adaptive and rational substitutes (Beck, Rush, Shaw, & Emery, 1979; Meichenbaum, 1977). Cognitive therapy guides patients, first, in distinguishing between normative and pathological changes in sleep patterns, and, second, in alleviating excessive concerns about sleep loss and its impact on daytime functioning. Such concerns in themselves perpetuate the vicious cycle of insomnia, fear of sleeplessness, emotional arousal, and further sleep disturbances.

## Educational Component

The educational component involves the teaching of basic sleep hygiene principles. A variety of lifestyle and environmental factors can be detrimental to a good night's sleep. In this module, the effects of diet, exercise, substance use, light, noise, and temperature are reviewed. A series of clinical guidelines to safeguard against their interference with sleep is outlined. These principles are often a matter of common knowledge, but adherence to good sleep hygiene practices is generally poor among insomniacs (Lacks & Rotert, 1986). Although they are rarely the primary cause of insomnia, these factors can complicate the sleep problem and impede therapeutic progress. Thus, education plays an important role by promoting better sleep hygiene practices.


## Medication Withdrawal Component

Although an occasional hypnotic may be helpful for some people, a significant proportion of patients seeking insomnia treatment are already dependent on sleep medications. In most cases, unsupervised attempts to taper off the use of hypnotics may have been unsuccessful and led only to more severe sleep difficulties. This module provides a structured withdrawal schedule for gradually discontinuing the usage of sleeping aids. Its design and timing with the overall intervention are individualized and based on the type, dosage, and frequency of drug use; the patient's readiness to discontinue medication; and the presence of concomitant psychiatric or physical disorders. It is necessary to enlist the collaboration of a physician for planning the safest withdrawal schedule with minimal risks of medical complications.


## The Setting

An outpatient clinic is the typical setting in which this treatment is carried out. Despite the phenomenal growth of sleep disorders centers in the past 10 years, only a small proportion of them have yet integrated insomnia clinics within their centers. As a result, many insomniacs are still only evaluated at sleep clinics and then referred to other facilities for treatment. Psychologists, psychiatrists, and other mental health professionals would benefit from establishing consultation–liaison services with those centers that do not provide clinical treatment for insomnia. Although this protocol is primarily designed for delivery on an outpatient basis, it may also be adapted to the needs of inpatients living in chronic care facilities (e.g., nursing homes). A few studies have also documented the efficacy of nonpharmacological interventions for the management of insomnia on inpatient psychiatric units (Edinger, Lipper, & Wheeler, 1989; Morin et al., 1990; Tan et al., 1987). Treatment can then be initiated during a patient's hospital stay as long as outpatient follow-ups are scheduled upon discharge. Generalization of clinical gains beyond the treatment setting needs to be programmed, so that the patient has an opportunity to practice and consolidate newly learned skills in the home environment.

# The Patient

The typical insomnia patient at our clinic comes in with a long-standing history of problems falling asleep and/or trouble staying asleep, along with complaints of daytime sequelae (e.g., fatigue, impaired performance, or mood disturbances). There are about two women for every one man seeking help for insomnia, and the age range varies widely from young adulthood to late life. More than 50% of the patients presenting in our clinic are habitual users of sleeping aids; a significant number also present with concomitant medical or psychological disorders. Although this program has been designed mostly for those with primary insomnias (i.e., psychophysiological, subjective, and idiopathic), preliminary findings indicate that it may benefit even patients whose insomnia is associated with chronic illnesses (Cannici, Malcolm, & Peek, 1983; Morin, Kowatch, & Wade, 1989), some patients with psychopathology (Morin et al., 1990; Tan et al., 1987), and patients with dependency on hypnotics (Morin et al., 1990). There is also ample evidence that older adults, those most at risk for insomnia, can benefit to a significant degree from this program (Morin, Kowatch, et al., 1993).

This intervention is not for individuals whose transient insomnia is secondary to acute and severe physical illnesses (e.g., acute pain) or major psychopathology (e.g., bipolar disorder in the manic phase). Pharmacotherapy is often the best and only alternative in these cases, though concurrent behavioral interventions may prevent the development of persistent insomnia. Behavior therapy may also prove a useful adjunct for sleep disturbances in the chronically mentally ill, but there are few specific outcome data on this population. Patients whose insomnia is attributable to circadian factors (e.g., jet lag, work shift, phase-delay or phase-advance syndromes) may be better candidates for alternative therapies (e.g., light therapy), though when the insomnia is chronic they may also benefit from psychological interventions, inasmuch as behavioral and cognitive factors are involved in perpetuating the sleep problem. Patients whose insomnia is secondary to mild sleep apnea or periodic leg movements may benefit from this approach, but in the more severe cases treatment must focus on the primary sleep disorders.

It is important during the initial evaluation to ascertain whether sleep is the patient's chief concern. Because insomnia is more socially acceptable than other dysfunctions (e.g., depression), a person may be more inclined to acknowledge sleep problems and may flatly deny the presence of other difficulties, which may in fact be the main motivation for seeking counseling. Likewise, some individuals involved in a dysfunctional marital relationship may focus exclusively on sleep disturbances and systematically ignore the marital problems. These clinical issues deserve careful consideration before treatment is initiated.

In summary, this treatment protocol has been developed specifically for individuals whose insomnia has become chronic and out of control, and for whom sleeping without drugs is a desirable and realistic goal. Psychological and medical factors can contribute to sleep disturbances, but the severity and time course of these concurrent problems should determine the initial treatment focus. The basic philosophy of this program is that a time-limited intervention focusing directly on the perpetuating factors may prove useful, regardless of the initial precipitating conditions. There is little if any empirical evidence supporting the use of symptom-specific interventions, and unless it is clear that insomnia is only one among several depressive symptoms, it is best to treat the sleep component directly. A case in point is that sleep disturbances in depressed patients often persist long after the depression has lifted (Hauri, Chernik, Hawkins, & Mendels, 1974).

## Duration of Treatment

The complete protocol involves one or two evaluation sessions and eight therapy sessions spread over a 10-week period. The first two sessions are devoted to clinical assessment by means of a detailed sleep history, a functional analysis of controlling variables, and a screening of concomitant physical and psychological problems (see Chapter 5). There is a 2-week self-monitoring period during which baseline data on the current sleep pattern are collected. At a minimum, eight therapy sessions are needed thereafter to implement all procedures, to promote maximum adherence to the regimen, and to build up self-management skills for coping with periodic insomnia likely to reoccur after treatment completion.

After the evaluation process is completed, therapy sessions are scheduled on a weekly basis. Because of extensive night-to-night variability in insomniacs' sleep patterns, this has proved the best timing for implementing the complete package. This schedule gives patients ample time to experiment with the newly introduced procedures, yet ensures continuity between sessions. When depressive or anxiety-related symptomatology is present, it may be preferable to hold the first few sessions closer to one another. Similarly, if steady progress is made toward the middle of treatment, the sessions may be spaced on a biweekly basis. Booster sessions are occasionally scheduled for patients whose self-efficacy remains low, despite significant sleep improvements after completion of the intervention.

It may be necessary to extend treatment duration beyond the customary 10-week period for several types of patients. For those who present with a long-standing history of medication use (i.e., those who are drug-dependent), treatment length varies according to the type, frequency, and duration of prior use and is also a function of patients' acceptance of and compliance with the intervention. When insomnia is associated with psychological (e.g., anxiety, depression) or medical conditions (e.g., chronic pain), treatment may last significantly longer than the suggested 8–10 weeks if these problems are addressed simultaneously. Unless it is clear that insomnia is strictly secondary in nature, we generally treat the sleep component first and only subsequently address these concomitant dysfunctions or refer the patients elsewhere.

## Format of Treatment

This intervention can be implemented either individually or in a group format (five to seven people). In addition to its cost-effectiveness, group therapy offers several advantages (Lacks, 1987, 1991). First, the opportunity to share a problem with others and to realize that one is not alone can be of great comfort. The group forum serves as a powerful social support network and alleviates some of the concerns surrounding the sleep problem. Second, model patients who diligently adhere to the clinical procedures can prove strong allies to the therapist in convincing other patients to comply with the prescribed regimen. Third, the group format may be a powerful deterrent to bringing up personal problems that are not directly relevant to sleep difficulties. The clinician can take advantage of this social inhibition factor to keep the therapy focused.

It is not always possible or desirable to treat insomnia patients in a group. Unless one has a specialized insomnia clinic or recruits persons with specific dysfunctions, it may be difficult to gather a sufficient number of patients at a given time to run group therapy. Some patients may simply prefer to be seen individually, or the clinician may decide that a patient's incidental psychopathology is severe enough that it would interfere with the group process. The clinical guidelines provided in the remaining chapters apply to both individual and group therapy unless otherwise specified.

## Structure and Length of Sessions

The treatment sessions last 50–60 minutes for individual therapy and 90 minutes for group therapy. These time limitations are stated explicitly to patients, in order to encourage promptness for scheduled appointments and to minimize the risk that some patients may be offended if the therapist needs to redirect attention. Each therapy session is well structured and covers a different facet of treatment. Although their specific content varies, most sessions are organized around six activities:

1. *Reviewing the sleep diary and progress from the previous week.* The very first item on the agenda is to review the sleep diary for the previous week. This quickly communicates the importance of self-monitoring. It is essential

to reinforce the patient verbally for bringing in the diary and for diligent monitoring, as this task may become aversive for some individuals over time. The patient is asked first to summarize his or her sleep pattern for that particular week; this offers an opportunity to observe possible dysfunctional cognitive processes. Then the therapist reviews the diary and simply states the facts about difficulties falling asleep or maintaining sleep for the previous week without doing any problem solving yet.

2. *Identifying problems encountered in home practice.* The next step consists of determining whether the patient understood and registered the clinical procedures previously described and whether he or she has complied with them. For several of the stimulus control and sleep restriction procedures, compliance can be gauged simply by examining the diary (e.g., bedtime, arising time). For other procedures (e.g., getting out of bed, sleep-incompatible behaviors), it is necessary to rely on the patient's verbal report. The patient is first asked to summarize his or her understanding of what was supposed to be done and the rationale for doing it. The next inquiry is whether he or she indeed complied with the recommendations. To enhance the learning process, each and every procedure should be reviewed weekly; the time spent on this task should decrease as the intervention unfolds. Most people do not comply with all procedures, but instead select only a few of them. The therapist must keep this possibility in mind continually.

3. *Designing and negotiating strategies for better treatment adherence.* After problems regarding adherence are identified, the next step consists of exploring underlying motivations, obstacles, and possible solutions to these problems. Because these issues will vary with each therapy component, I discuss them in more detail in the following chapters.

4. *Introducing the new treatment component and its rationale.* Once these problems have been resolved, a new treatment component is introduced. Each procedure is described along with its rationale and objectives. Clinical examples are provided for illustrative purposes. The patient is asked to summarize his or her understanding of the newly introduced therapy component.

5. *Presenting supportive didactic material.* As each therapy component is introduced, supportive didactic material may be used to reinforce the newly learned material. Some people may not readily integrate all information or theoretical foundations supporting a particular procedure. Handouts written for the layperson are helpful to consolidate information covered during a given session. The patient is asked to read them between sessions and to bring up questions at the following meeting. They are particularly helpful during the course of treatment, and also as a future reference for people who may encounter periodic relapses.

6. *Reviewing the homework assignment.* During the last segment of the session, the patient is asked to summarize homework assignments for the

following week. Corrective feedback is provided by the therapist when necessary. Each session concludes with a preview of materials to be covered at the
next visit.

## Outlines of Therapy Sessions

A session-by-session overview of the treatment protocol is presented in Table
6.1. An outline of each therapy session is also provided at the end of this
chapter. These outlines highlight the most important issues to be covered
during each session; lists of materials needed and reminders for the therapist
are also included. The specific content of each session is discussed in more
detail in later chapters. These outlines tell the reader where to find the
material needed for each session.

Parts of the first two sessions are devoted to assessment. With the
Insomnia Interview Schedule (Appendix A), a detailed history of the insomnia problem is obtained, and a careful functional analysis of its controlling variables is conducted. Sleep diary monitoring (Appendix F) is initiated to
obtain baseline data. Several psychometric instruments are administered to
evaluate the presence of concomitant mood disturbances and/or psychopathology (see Chapter 5 for details). The Sleep Impairment Index
(Appendix B), Beliefs and Attitudes about Sleep Scale (Appendix C), and the
Insomnia Treatment Acceptability Scale (Appendix D) are also administered.
One session may be enough to conduct this initial assessment, but a second

TABLE 6.1. Outline of Insomnia Treatment Protocol

| Session | Activities |
| --- | --- |
| | *Assessment* |
| 1–2 | Insomnia Interview Schedule, baseline sleep diary monitoring, psychological screening, Beliefs and Attitudes about Sleep Scale, Sleep Impairment Index, Insomnia Treatment Acceptability Scale, and optional polysomnography |
| | *Treatment* |
| 1 | Program overview; social learning explanation of insomnia; goal setting and behavioral contract; initiation of medication withdrawal (see text) |
| 2–3 | Behavioral component: Stimulus control instructions and sleep restriction therapy |
| 4–5 | Cognitive component: Cognitive restructuring |
| 6 | Educational component: Sleep hygiene |
| 7 | Review and integration of all therapy components; design of methods for promoting adherence; programming generalization of newly learned skills |
| 8 | Identification of high-risk situations; review of relapse prevention strategies; further consolidation of therapeutic gains |

session is often necessary when medical or psychological complicating factors are present.

*Treatment Session 1.* An overview of the treatment program is presented during the first therapy session. Each therapy component is briefly introduced, but the actual procedures are not described yet. The agenda of the following seven sessions is reviewed. The therapist introduces the self-management approach, and a conceptual model of insomnia is reviewed. Figure 4.1 is used to illustrate how situational insomnia evolves into a chronic problem over time, whereas Figure 4.2 is used to depict the vicious cycle of anxiety, insomnia, more arousal, and further sleep disturbances. Basic facts about the nature of sleep and about some changes occurring over the course of the lifespan are presented. This information is mostly extracted from Chapter 2. At the end of the session, the goal-setting form is completed jointly by the clinician and patient, and the personal contract (Appendix E) is signed.

*Treatment Session 2.* The behavioral therapy component is introduced during the second session. The sleep restriction and stimulus control procedures are described along with their rationales (see Chapter 8). The patient's resistance and obstacles to implementing these procedures are discussed briefly, but the patient is encouraged to experiment with these procedures first and to bring up problems at the next session.

*Treatment Session 3.* This session is mostly devoted to problem-solving difficulties encountered in the first week of home practice. Each procedure is reviewed, and the patient is prompted for whether he or she complied with it or not. Specific methods to enhance treatment adherence are reviewed. The initial "sleep window" is revised, and allowable time in bed is modified according to the guidelines discussed in chapter 8.

*Treatment Session 4.* The cognitive therapy component is introduced in this session. The basic principles, goals, and rationale of cognitive restructuring are discussed (see Chapter 9). The relevance of this framework for understanding insomnia is highlighted. After the initial groundwork has been done, 4 of the 12 clinical vignettes presented in Chapter 9 are reviewed. These are derived from the Beliefs and Attitudes about Sleep Scale. Following the three-step model (identify, challenge, correct), the therapist selects those vignettes most clinically relevant to the patient, examines their validity, and then guides the patient in replacing them with more adaptive substitutes. One vignette for each theme (causal attributions, expectations, etc.) is addressed during this session. The patient is instructed to monitor sleep-related self-statements during the upcoming week.

*Treatment Session 5.* After issues related to compliance with the behavioral procedures are reviewed, this session continues with cognitive therapy. Four additional vignettes from Chapter 9 are selected, with one from each theme (attributions, control, catastrophizing, etc.). Additional dysfunctional cognitions monitored by the patient in the preceding week are reviewed, and if judged dysfunctional, they are replaced with more adaptive substitutes. At this stage of treatment, progress made toward goal attainment is discussed with the patient by reviewing the summary data sheet (Appendix G).

*Treatment Session 6.* Sleep hygiene education (see Chapter 10) is discussed in this session. The following items are reviewed to determine and safeguard against their interference with sleep: caffeine, nicotine, alcohol, diet, exercise, noise, light, and room temperature. The main objectives are to teach and promote healthier sleep hygiene practices. The last four vignettes of the cognitive therapy module are also reviewed in this session, as well as other dysfunctional cognitions monitored by the patient in the preceding week. Continued adherence to stimulus control and sleep restriction procedures is checked, and alteration in allowable time in bed is made as needed.

*Treatment Session 7.* In this session the clinician reviews all therapy components in an integrated fashion. Feedback regarding progress made is provided, and areas that need particular attention are highlighted. Process–outcome relationships are examined. The "sleep window" is adjusted so that actual time spent in bed is brought closer to the patient's goal. Methods for promoting continued adherence to this multifaceted intervention are reviewed.

*Treatment Session 8.* In this last session strategies for preventing or minimizing relapse are presented. High-risk situations are identified, and the patient is taught strategies to prevent or minimize sleep disturbances in those situations. Coping skills to deal with residual sleep disturbances and with the inevitable occasional poor night's sleep is reviewed. The main objective is to prevent such reactions as catastrophizing, overgeneralization, or selective focus, which in the past have contributed to setting the stage for chronic insomnia.

The specific content of each session is discussed in greater detail in the following chapters. The sequence of therapy components may be altered as needed. For example, if excessive caffeine intake is a salient contributing factor, it may be necessary to implement the educational component first, because sleep improvements may be impeded otherwise. When sleep medication is involved to the extent that it is judged to be part of the problem, withdrawal from such medication can be introduced at any time during the course of the intervention. Although it is generally desirable to begin decreasing medication intake early (e.g., session 3), a patient's readiness, anxiety level, and self-efficacy often determine the most appropriate timing for introducing this component. More details about these issues are provided in Chapter 11. Finally, the clinician should feel free to use other procedures that are not included in the treatment protocol described here (see Hauri, 1991). Although there is no clear evidence that matching insomnia patients to specific treatment modalities produces better outcomes, some individuals may benefit from the complementary use of relaxation-based procedures. These issues are discussed further in Chapter 12.

## Treatment Session 1

1. Self-monitoring
   a. Review sleep diary
   b. Answer questions pertaining to diary only
   c. Reinforce patient for self-monitoring

2. Program overview
   a. Behavioral: Changing maladaptive sleep habits
   b. Cognitive: Reframing dysfunctional beliefs and attitudes
   c. Educational: Promoting good sleep hygiene practices
   d. Medication: Planning a schedule to discontinue sleep aids

3. Agenda of therapy sessions 1–8

4. Nature of self-management approach
   a. Emphasize the notion of self-control and problem-solving skills
   b. Contrast this approach with dependency upon sleeping pills
   c. Stress the active role of patient in treatment process
   d. Discuss the time-limited format of the intervention program

5. Social learning explanation of insomnia
   a. Describe contributing factors: predisposing, precipitating, perpetuating factors
   b. Review conceptual model of insomnia (see Figures 4.1 and 4.2)
   c. Relate this model to the patient's personal sleep problem history

6. Basic facts about sleep and changes in sleep patterns over the lifespan
   a. The nature of sleep (stages 1–4 NREM, REM)
   b. Prevalence of insomnia and sociodemographic correlates
   c. Changes in sleep patterns over the course of the lifespan

7. Goal setting and personal contract

**Materials:**
Sleep diary (Appendix F)
Figures 4.1 and 4.2

**Reminders:**
Importance of self-monitoring
No self-initiated changes

## Treatment Session 2

1. Self-monitoring
   a. Review sleep diary
   b. Answer questions pertaining to diary only
   c. Reinforce patient for self-monitoring

2. Introduction of behavioral (sleep restriction and stimulus control) procedures
   a. Restrict time in bed to ___ hours per night
   b. Optional daytime naps (<1 hour) no later than 3 P.M.
   c. Go to bed only when sleepy
   d. Get out of bed when unable to fall asleep/return to sleep within 10–15 minutes.
   e. Repeat this procedure as often as necessary
   f. Arise at the same time every morning
   g. Do not use the bed/bedroom for nonsleeping activities

3. Treatment rationale

**Materials:**                                    **Reminders:**
Sleep diary (Appendix F)                          Importance of self-monitoring
Goal-setting form (Table 7.1)                      Time-limited format
Handout on behavioral procedures (Table 8.1)
Personal contract (Appendix E)

## Treatment Session 3

1. Self-monitoring
   a. Review sleep diary
   b. Answer questions pertaining to diary only
   c. Reinforce participants for self-monitoring

2. Review of behavioral procedures and their rationale
   a. Restrict time in bed to __ hours per night
   b. Optional daytime naps (<1 hour) no later than 3 P.M.
   c. Go to bed only when sleepy
   d. Get out of bed when unable to fall asleep/return to sleep within 10–15 minutes.
   e. Repeat this procedure as often as necessary
   f. Arise at the same time every morning
   g. Do not use the bed/bedroom for nonsleeping activities

3. Review of problems encountered in home practice

4. Generation of methods to enhance compliance
   a. Find activities to engage in when getting out of bed
   b. Identify cues to determine sleepiness and time to return to bed
   c. Use alarm clock to maintain regular arising time
   d. Find competing activities to fight urge to take nap or overwhelming sleepiness before prescribed bedtime
   e. Secure support from spouse/significant others
   f. Remember the time-limited format of program
   g. Pace activity levels and change their timing

5. Review of homework assignment and sleep window (restriction of time in bed)

6. Preview of session 4—cognitive therapy

**Material:**
Sleep diary (Appendix F)

**Reminders:**
Importance of self-monitoring
Time-limited format

## Treatment Session 4

1. Self-monitoring
   a. Review sleep diary
   b. Answer questions pertaining to diary only
   c. Reinforce participants for self-monitoring

2. Review of home practice and problems with behavioral procedures
   a. Restrict time in bed to __ hours per night
   b. Optional daytime naps (<1 hour) no later than 3 P.M.
   c. Go to bed only when sleepy
   d. Get out of bed when unable to fall asleep/return to sleep within 10–15 mininutes.
   e. Repeat this procedure as often as necessary
   f. Arise at the same time every morning
   g. Do not use the bed/bedroom for nonsleeping activities

3. Enhancing compliance with treatment requirements
   a. Find activities to engage in when getting out of bed
   b. Find competing activities to fight sleepiness at inappropriate times
   c. Secure support from spouse/significant others
   d. Use alarm clock to maintain regular arising time
   e. Identify behavioral cues of sleepiness (yawning, heavier eyelids)

4. Cognitive therapy
   a. Introduce basic principles, rationale, and goals of cognitive therapy
   b. Discuss clinical relevance of this framework with regard to insomnia
   c. Select four vignettes from Chapter 9
   d. Identify, challenge, and replace dysfunctional cognitions
      i. Correct misconceptions about the causes of insomnia
      ii. Alter dysfunctional beliefs about the impact of insomnia
      iii. Modify unrealistic sleep expectations
      iv. Enhance perceptions of control and predictability
      v. Dispel myths about good sleep practices
   e. Generate additional patient-specific maladaptive self-statements

**Materials:**
Sleep diary (Appendix F)
Beliefs and Attitudes about Sleep Scale (Appendix C)
Clinical vignettes (Chapter 9)
Handout on sleep cognitions and affect (Table 9.1)

**Reminder:**
Time-limited format

## Treatment Session 5

1. Self-monitoring
   a. Review sleep diary
   b. Answer questions pertaining to diary only
   c. Reinforce participants for self-monitoring

2. Review of home practice and problems with behavioral procedures
   a. Restrict time in bed to __ hours per night
   b. Optional daytime naps (<1 hour) no later than 3 P.M.
   c. Go to bed only when sleepy
   d. Get out of bed when unable to fall asleep/return to sleep within 10–15 mininutes.
   e. Repeat this procedure as often as necessary
   f. Arise at the same time every morning
   g. Do not use the bed/bedroom for nonsleeping activities

3. Cognitive therapy
   a. Review principles, rationale, and goals of cognitive therapy
   b. Discuss clinical relevance of this framework with regard to insomnia
   c. Select four more vignettes from Chapter 9
   d. Identify, challenge, and replace dysfunctional cognitions
      i. Correct misconceptions about the causes of insomnia
      ii. Alter dysfunctional beliefs about the impact of insomnia
      iii. Modify unrealistic sleep expectations
      iv. Enhance perceptions of control and predictability
      v. Dispel myths about good sleep practices
   e. Generate additional patient-specific maladaptive self-statements

4. Review of progress and goal attainment

5. Preview of session 6—sleep hygiene education

**Materials:**
Sleep diary (Appendix F)
Summary data sheet and goal-setting form (Appendix G, Table 7.1)
Beliefs and Attitudes about Sleep Scale (Appendix C)
Clinical vignettes (Chapter 9)

## Treatment Session 6

1. Self-monitoring
   a. Review sleep diary
   b. Answer questions pertaining to diary only
   c. Reinforce patient for self-monitoring

2. Review of home practice and problems with behavioral procedures
   a. Restrict time in bed to __ hours per night
   b. Optional daytime naps (<1 hour) no later than 3 P.M.
   c. Go to bed only when sleepy
   d. Get out of bed when unable to fall asleep/return to sleep within 10–15 minutes.
   e. Repeat this procedure as often as necessary
   f. Arise at the same time every morning
   g. Do not use the bed/bedroom for nonsleeping activities

3. Cognitive therapy
   a. Select additional vignettes from Chapter 9 and from patient self-monitoring forms
   b. Replace dysfunctional cognitions
      i. Correct misconceptions about the causes of insomnia
      ii. Alter dysfunctional beliefs about the impact of insomnia
      iii. Modify unrealistic sleep expectations
      iv. Enhance perceptions of control and predictability
      v. Dispel myths about good sleep practices

4. Sleep hygiene education
   a. Caffeine
   b. Nicotine
   c. Alcohol
   d. Diet
   e. Exercise
   f. Noise, light, temperature

**Materials:**                                                    **Reminder:**
Sleep diary (Appendix F)                                          Time-limited format
Sleep hygiene handout (Table 10.1)
Beliefs and Attitudes about Sleep Scale (Appendix C)
Clinical vignettes (Chapter 9)

## Treatment Session 7

1. Self-monitoring
   a. Review sleep diary
   b. Answer questions pertaining to diary only
   c. Reinforce patient for self-monitoring
2. Answering questions and resolving problems regarding sleep hygiene principles
3. Brief review and integration of all therapy components
4. Feedback to patient
   a. Provide feedback regarding progress and compliance with treatment
   b. Emphasize specific problem areas that need more attention
   c. Examine process and outcome relationships
   d. Increase time in bed so that it gets closer to baseline values
5. Review of behavioral procedures
   a. Restrict time in bed to __ hours per night
   b. Optional daytime naps (<1 hour) no later than 3 P.M.
   c. Go to bed only when sleepy
   d. Get out of bed when unable to fall asleep/return to sleep within 10–15 minutes.
   e. Repeat this procedure as often as necessary
   f. Arise at the same time every morning
   g. Do not use the bed/bedroom for nonsleeping activities

**Materials:**
Sleep diary (Appendix F)
Summary data sheet and goal-setting form (Appendix G, Table 7.1)

## Treatment Session 8

1.  Self-monitoring (see previous session outlines)
2.  Brief review and integration of all treatment procedures
3.  Maintaining treatment gains
    a. Motivation and commitment
    b. Continued adherence to treatment (making it part of one's lifestyle)
    c. Social support from spouse or significant others
4.  Relapse prevention
    a. Make distinction among lapse, relapse, and collapse
    b. Discuss the inevitability of having an occasional poor night's sleep and caution against interpreting this as evidence that chronic insomnia has returned
    c. Identify high-risk situations
        i. Negative emotional states (e.g., stress, anxiety, depression)
        ii. Positive emotional states (e.g., anticipation of a trip, baby)
    d. Give tips for coping with the inevitable
        i. Stay calm—no need to panic, it just makes things worse
        ii. Analyze antecedents or precipitating circumstances
        iii. Reinstate restriction of time in bed and follow stimulus control procedures
        iv. Ask for further help—phone call, booster session
    e. Give tips for coping with daytime sequelae of insomnia
        i. Change the timing of scheduled activities
        ii. Engage in sensory stimulation and time management to increase performance
        iii. Increase tolerance to sleep loss
5.  Review of progress and goal attainment

**Materials:**
Sleep diary (Appendix F)
Summary data sheet and goal-setting form
(Appendix G, Table 7.1)

**Reminder:**
Booster sessions

# 7

## Preparing the Patient for Treatment

This chapter describes several preparatory steps needed to enlist the patient's collaboration in the therapeutic process. Most individuals seeking insomnia treatment are not familiar with the underlying principles of cognitive-behavioral therapy, and it is essential to prepare them accordingly. The following topics are covered: self-management principles, the patient's expectations and treatment acceptance, record keeping, therapy goals, contract negotiation, and securing support from significant others. Failure to address these issues right from the start may hinder compliance and progress; worse, it may lead to treatment failure. This material is usually discussed at the end of the evaluation or during the very first therapy session.

### Introducing the Self-Management Approach

The first task for the therapist is to introduce the self-management approach and its basic principles. The cornerstone of this approach, which is common to most cognitive-behavioral therapies, is that the patient assumes an active role in his or her treatment. As such, the patient is encouraged to develop a "personal scientist" attitude and to take control of his or her own destiny. This means increasing his or her awareness or insight into the sleep problem and its controlling factors. It is only after gaining a better understanding of the causes and effects of insomnia that the patient can learn self-management skills to alter these controlling variables.

The therapist's role is one of facilitator and problem solver. He or she is actively engaged in the therapeutic process by providing specific guidelines, instructions, and corrective feedback. A directive approach is adopted, therapy is task-oriented, and the focus is on teaching the patient problem-solving skills to minimize sleep difficulties and to cope with any residual insomnia after completion of treatment. As such, the main emphasis is not on curing insomnia, but rather on developing appropriate coping skills. The procedures are described within a self-control framework in which the patient is responsible for implementation. Unlike a more traditional model in which a patient is simply a passive recipient of treatment, here nothing is done to or for him or her; the patient does it. As in most brief therapies, it is essential to establish a collaborative working relationship between the clinician and the patient (Garfield, 1989). Along with genuine empathy and support, a strong thera-pist–patient alliance is necessary, because much of the treatment depends upon the patient's willingness to carry out therapeutic instructions (Bootzin, 1985). The ultimate goal, however, is to foster the patient's independence and self-control.

It should be made clear early that this intervention is a highly structured regimen; time, effort, and diligent adherence to homework assignments are required if sleep is to improve. This cannot be overemphasized. Although some procedures may initially appear simplistic and straightforward, the patient should be cautioned that regular and consistent adherence to the entire program is the key to a successful outcome. Indeed, one of the main reasons for holding weekly sessions is to facilitate treatment adherence and provide ongoing feedback. Supplementary didactic material is most helpful, but bibliotherapy alone is rarely sufficient for the management of chronic insomnia.

It is often necessary to contrast this self-management approach with more traditional methods—those that involve routine sleeping pill pre-scriptions or behavior change recommendations without any systematic fol-low-up. Some chronic insomniacs are used to a monthly visit to a primary care physician for a refill of hypnotics. These visits are usually brief, lasting 5 to 10 minutes; worse, prescriptions are renewed over the phone. There is little attempt at directly solving sleep problems, and these symptomatic in-terventions often lead to frustrations and continued difficulties. It is essential to point out that there is no such "quick fix" for chronic insomnia. The time frame for implementing the present program is discussed right at the onset. To avoid premature termination, the patient is cautioned that no miracle cure should be expected in one or two office visits. A time commitment of at least 10 weeks is required; this time-limited format is emphasized to maximize compliance. Considering that most patients have suffered from insomnia for years, this represents a very short investment of time.

## Gauging the Patient's Expectations

Chronic insomniacs come to therapy with various backgrounds in terms of insomnia history, prior exposure to treatment, and current expectations. These variables may have a significant impact on subsequent treatment adherence and outcome and should be explored early (see Chambers, 1992). Despite their widespread prevalence, sleep complaints often remain untreated for years (Mellinger et al., 1985). Several reasons may explain this paradox. First, people may assume that sleeping pills are the only treatment available, yet many people may prefer to endure sleep disturbances rather than having to rely on medication. Second, insomnia is not as lethal or painful as other disorders (e.g., depression), and it does not affect significant others to the same extent as a substance abuse problem may. Finally, many people attempt to cure insomnia with a variety of self-remedies (e.g., a hot bath, herbal tea, over-the-counter sleep aids), and the intermittent success of these interventions may delay their seeking professional help.

The following statements exemplify the diversity of patients' initial expectations:

> "I didn't know anything could be done for insomnia until I read this article in the newspaper."
> "I don't believe much can be done about this problem, but I am willing to try anything."
> "I have tried it all and nothing works."

Many individuals with chronic and untreated sleep problems have developed overly pessimistic attitudes, believing that insomnia has just become a fact of life. Others come to therapy with overly optimistic expectations, and their only goal is to cure this sleep problem forever. It is important to convey a sense of hope and to model a positive yet realistic attitude regarding outcome. At the same time, it is advisable to minimize exclusive focus on curing the sleep problem. Instead, regaining control and learning new skills for coping with an occasional poor night's sleep, which plagues virtually everyone at one time or another, should be emphasized. As Bootzin (1985) has cogently noted, a most important goal of insomnia treatment is to alter a patient's view that he or she is a victim of the sleep problem to one in which he or she is capable of coping with the problem. It should be stressed that treatment is designed to improve self-management skills; as such, it involves changing daytime and nighttime behaviors, attitudes, and beliefs that interfere with sleep. As a final point, it is good clinical practice to inform the consumer about the efficacy of this intervention and the range of possible outcomes for patients presenting with similar sleep problem severity and history. The clinician can use the figures presented in Chapter 12 to discuss typical improvement rates obtained for sleep-onset latency, number and duration of awakenings, and total sleep time.

## Assessing Treatment Acceptability

Although pharmacotherapy is the most commonly used method for treating insomnia, the recent recognition and high publicity accorded to side effects (e.g., amnesia) of some sleep medications (e.g., Halcion) have raised concerns among potential consumers. On the other hand, there is much empirical evidence supporting the use of psychological interventions, but little is known about how acceptable these methods are to the public. Patients' attitudes toward treatment modality usually fall into one of three broad categories. Some insomniacs expect to be prescribed a drug, either because they are unaware of alternative treatments or unwilling to undergo such interventions. Others have very negative attitudes toward drugs and do not comply with prescribed sleep medications. Still others have become drug-dependent but wish to get off medication if an effective alternative is available. Because consumer acceptability and perceived effectiveness of a given intervention may affect compliance and thereby outcome, it is important to address these social validation issues (Kazdin, 1986).

My colleagues and I have developed a measure designed to evaluate patients' acceptance of psychological and pharmacological therapies for insomnia. The Insomnia Treatment Acceptability Scale (Appendix D) briefly describes two treatment methods commonly used for insomnia. The psychological treatment is described as a self-management program aimed at changing poor sleep habits, regulating sleep schedules, and altering dysfunctional thoughts about insomnia. The pharmacological treatment is described as a new sleeping pill designed to induce sleep by reducing physiological and cognitive arousal at bedtime. Both therapies are described as equally effective methods. After reading each description, the patient completes nine ratings on visual analogue scales. These ratings cover issues of treatment acceptance, intent to comply, perceived suitability for sleep-onset and sleep-maintenance problems, and expected effectiveness and side effects. To minimize the effects of demand characteristics, this measure is administered before the patient is exposed to any treatment material, preferably during the initial evaluation. This instrument provides useful information about the patient's attitudes toward and expectations of prospective interventions.

Among insomniacs recruited for outcome research, the psychological intervention is perceived as more acceptable and more suitable; it is also expected to be more effective in the long term and to produce fewer side effects than pharmacotherapy (Morin, Gaulier, et al., 1992). It is unclear, however, whether these results would generalize to individuals spontaneously seeking treatment in various clinical settings. Thus, much preparatory work may need to be done with those expecting to receive drug treatment and having an unfavorable attitude toward a more time-consuming behavioral management program. It is necessary to remind those patients that most hypnotic drugs produce rapid but sometimes short-lived sleep relief. In contrast, psychological methods may take a little longer to yield improvement, but these benefits are usually longer-lasting.

## Keeping a Sleep Diary

Maintaining a daily sleep diary is an essential requirement of this program, and this should be made clear during the initial evaluation. The sleep diary is an important therapeutic tool to document initial problem severity, progress, night-to-night variations in sleep patterns, and compliance with the clinical procedures. It is very difficult to run an effective therapy session when a patient fails to monitor his or her sleep or forgets to bring in the diary. The patient should view the diary as a "ticket" to get into the weekly therapy sessions. Noncompliance with self-monitoring is indicative of noncompliance with subsequent clinical recommendations.

Guidelines for coding the sleep diary are described in Chapter 5. Here the clinician re-emphasizes the importance of good and timely record keeping. There is no need for the patient to watch the clock constantly to provide exact times; only estimates of the sleep parameters are needed. It is not so much absolute accuracy (which is almost impossible to attain) as daily recording that is important. If self-monitoring is overlooked on a particular day, patients should be discouraged from going back and estimating sleep parameters retrospectively. Sleep diary data are entered into a summary form, which is periodically reviewed throughout treatment.

## Setting Goals

Most insomnia sufferers seeking therapy want to sleep longer and enjoy better sleep quality. It is important to define these global goals in more discrete and operational terms. People attach very different meanings to the concept of "a good night's sleep." For some, it means long sleep; for others, it means uninterrupted sleep; for still others, it means deep sleep. Sleep quality is difficult to define and does not always correlate with sleep duration or with the amount of time spent in a given sleep stage (e.g., stages 3–4). Goal setting is useful to keep the therapy focused; it keeps the therapist–patient alliance task-oriented and minimizes diversion to irrelevant materials. It also provides useful data about the patient's sleep expectations. Cognitive restructuring will prove useful in altering unrealistic expectations.

After the initial baseline period, the patient sets goals he or she would like to achieve by the end of treatment. Specific values are entered on a goal-setting form (Table 7.1) for each of the four main sleep parameters and, if applicable, for medication intake. The section "Current sleep pattern" is completed first by entering the baseline data. For example, sleep-onset latency may have averaged 60 minutes per night, with a total sleep time of 6 hours per night during this period. If for some reasons these 2 weeks are not representative of the patient's typical sleep pattern, extending the baseline duration is desirable, though this option is often impractical in clinical practice. Goals for each parameter are then entered in the section "Desired sleep pattern." The goal-setting form can be customized. Additional indices of sleep quality and daytime functioning, though more difficult to define, may be added to the quantitative variables.

Selecting goals that are acceptable to patients is important, but these goals must also be attainable rather than too idealistic. For example, if a person wishes to fall asleep within 5 minutes of turning out the lights, the clinician may need to negotiate a somewhat more realistic objective. Likewise, a mean sleep-onset latency of 20–30 minutes does not leave much room for improvement. The therapist needs to modify these unrealistic expectations either now or later in treatment. Explaining that 30 minutes is the typical cutoff value to determine the clinical significance of sleep-onset insomnia may lower such expectations and diminish concerns about being unable to fall asleep more quickly. Some people wish that they could sleep uninterrupted for 8 hours, because they have been led to believe that this is the magic number that everyone should aim for. Therapy goals should be individualized, and the patient should be made aware that there is no "gold standard" for sleep duration; one should only aim for the number of hours that is needed to subjectively feel refreshed in the morning and function well during the day. The important point is to maximize success and minimize failure. When the patient's goals appear unrealistic, the clinician can negotiate them at this time or wait to address their appropriateness with cognitive restructuring techniques. Regardless of the alternative selected, therapy goals often need to be re-evaluated and readjusted periodically as the intervention unfolds.

**TABLE 7.1.** Goal-Setting Form

| | |
|---|---|
| *Current sleep pattern* (before treatment) | |
| Based on a typical night's sleep (i.e., past 2 weeks), how long does it take you to fall asleep after turning the lights off? | ____ minutes |
| How many times do you wake up in the middle of the night? | ____ times |
| How much time do you typically spend awake in the middle of the night? (total duration for all awakenings combined) | ____ minutes |
| On a typical night, how many hours of sleep do you get? | ____ hours |
| How many nights per week do you use a sleep aid? | ____ nights |
| *Desired sleep pattern* (after completing treatment) | |
| After turning the lights off, I would like to fall asleep in . . . | ____ minutes |
| If I still wake up in the middle of the night after treatment, I would like to wake up no more than . . . | ____ times |
| If I still wake up in the middle of the night after treatment, I would like to be awake for no more than . . . | ____ minutes |
| If I still wake up too early in the morning, I would like to wake up no more than ____ minutes before the desired time. | ____ minutes |
| I need this much sleep to feel rested and function well during the day and would like to achieve this sleep duration: | ____ hours |
| I would like to use sleep aids no more than ____ nights per week. | ____ nights |

It is sometimes necessary to have a secondary set of goals targeting procedures rather than outcome. This is particularly useful in dealing with noncompliance. A useful strategy is to write a behavioral contract setting explicit rules and contingencies for adhering to record-keeping requirements and to clinical procedures (e.g., maintaining a specific bedtime and arising time, eliminating daytime napping).

## Negotiating a Time-Limited Contract

Behavioral contracting has proved an effective therapeutic adjunct in the management of several clinical dysfunctions. A somewhat less rigid contractual form is used in the current program. Entered into by the therapist and patient jointly, this personal contract (see Appendix E) does not involve exchanges of specific reinforcers between the parties involved. Rather, it states explicitly the terms of the therapy agreement, what is expected from the patient and from the therapist, and what time frame is involved. In some respects, it is more like a consent form than a true contingency contract. It may look "childish" to some, but such written agreements often foster compliance. It is presented as an opportunity for the patient to make a personal but formal commitment to follow through on the entire treatment program. When compliance is expected to be problematic, the contract's format may be altered, with specific terms and contingencies stated explicitly and reinforcing consequences built into the contractual agreement.

## Securing Support from Significant Others

This cognitive-behavioral intervention requires several changes in sleep habits, schedules, and lifestyles that are likely to affect not only patients but their spouses or partners as well. Securing support from significant others will greatly facilitate successful implementation. Although the involvement of spouses or partners is not required, they are invited to attend the second session when most behavioral procedures are introduced. If this proves impractical, they are encouraged to read the handouts that summarize the procedures and their rationale.

Obtaining the support of significant others is a good idea for several reasons. First, many couples enjoy reading or watching TV in bed around bedtime. Patients may need guidance to make assertive requests and negotiate compromises with their significant others in order to comply with treatment requirements, which may necessitate modifying bedtime routines, avoiding reading or watching TV in bed, or moving the TV out of the bedroom. If spouses or partners are made aware of the nature and goals of treatment, they are more likely to cooperate with the patients in these matters. Significant others can even serve as allies for promoting treatment adherence. They may interrupt patients caught napping or remind them to curtail sleep-incompatible behaviors.

Spouses or partners can also collaborate with data collection. We usually ask a significant other to independently complete a measure of sleep impairment similar to the one completed by the patient. This consists of several Likert-type ratings of (1) awareness of the patient's sleep problem; (2) perceived severity; (3) degree of interference with daytime functioning; and (4) noticeability of impairment attributable to the sleep problem (see Appendix B). Additional ratings of perceived improvement and compliance are added at posttreatment. These collateral ratings provide excellent indices of social validation of treatment outcome. A spouse or partner may be asked to independently monitor some sleep parameters (e.g., sleep-onset latency, time in bed). Such assistance is highly desirable for reliability check in outcome research, though in a clinical context it may raise negative feelings if a patient perceives that this is done to check on the accuracy of his or her subjective reports.

Finally, significant others can provide useful information about reinforcing contingencies maintaining sleep difficulties. Potential secondary gains should be carefully explored (Chambers, 1992), as noted in Chapter 5. Avoidance of sexual intimacy; escape from child care or household responsibilities; or sympathy from a spouse/partner, friends, or coworkers can serve as subtle reinforcers in maintaining insomnia. Whether a patient and his or her significant other share the same bed or bedroom or sleep in separate quarters may have important implications. Most people sleeping in a separate bedroom say they do so because they wish to avoid disturbing their significant others or because they are kept awake by loud snoring. Although these are legitimate reasons, they may also be a more acceptable way of avoiding intimacy. The therapist should inquire diligently about these factors. Systematic inquiry as to how a spouse or partner responds to a patient's sleep complaints and medication use may reveal useful information. This information may be gathered directly from patients, but somewhat divergent perspectives are occasionally presented by significant others. Their involvement in the evaluation process is helpful to determine whether they will prove good therapeutic allies or whether they may have a hidden agenda that could sabotage therapeutic efforts. Marital therapy may at times be indicated either in place of or concomitant to sleep therapy.

In summary, several preparatory steps must be taken before initiating treatment. Issues related to treatment, patient, and contextual variables are discussed "up front" to determine whether a patient is appropriate for the type of therapy outlined in this manual. It is essential to address these issues early in order to enlist the patient's collaboration in the therapeutic process, to maximize compliance, and to minimize premature termination.

# 8

## Behavioral Treatment Component

This chapter describes the first and probably the most important component of the insomnia treatment program—the behavioral module. It consists of a combination of stimulus control and sleep restriction procedures. These methods are designed to modify maladaptive behavioral practices that perpetuate the insomnia problem. After the etiological role of these maladaptive sleep habits is reviewed, the clinical procedures are described, along with their rationale, goals, and methods of implemention. Problematic issues likely to arise during the course of treatment are discussed, and recommendations to facilitate patient adherence to the prescribed regimen are outlined.

### Maladaptive Sleep Habits and Insomnia

Chronic insomnia does not develop overnight. Common precipitating events include personal losses, occupational stress, and marital conflict. Reactive anxiety or depression is the predominant contributing factor in the acute phase of insomnia. As the stressors fade away or individuals adjust to them, most people resume their normal sleep patterns. However, individuals who are more prone to insomnia or more susceptible to conditioning may develop negative responses to stimuli normally conducive to sleep (e.g., bed, bedtime, bedroom). What used to be the place and time for relaxation and sleep are now associated with arousal and sleeplessness. With repeated occurrences, a conditioning process evolves; the eventual result is a vicious cycle of insomnia, more arousal, and further sleep disturbances. Several maladaptive behavior patterns may also feed into the problem. The most common ones include maintaining irregular sleep schedules, napping routinely in the daytime, spending excessive amounts of time in bed, and using the bed or bedroom for nonsleeping activities. Not all insomniacs engaged in these practices to the same extent, and not all people who do so necessarily have sleep difficulties. However, many of these practices are used as coping strategies to deal with the debilitating effects of sleep disturbances. They may

**109**

temporarily help to compensate for sleep loss, but in the long run, they are instrumental in turning what might otherwise have been a transient insomnia problem into a persistent one. Eliminating these maladaptive behaviors is one of the most critical components in the management of chronic insomnia.

## Treatment Goals and Rationale

The behavior therapy component is aimed at achieving two goals: (1) to strengthen the association between sleep behaviors and such stimuli as the bed, bedtime, and the bedroom surroundings; and (2) to consolidate sleep over shorter periods of time spent in bed. The first goal is the object of stimulus control therapy, which is designed to eliminate both overt and covert sleep-incompatible activities. The second one is a function of sleep restriction, which curtails the amount of time spent in bed.

The rationale underlying the use of these procedures in the management of insomnia is that sleep is a behavior susceptible to conditioning processes to the same extent as waking behaviors are. Its occurrence at fairly regular intervals is partly governed by environmental and temporal stimuli. When the stimulus conditions normally conducive to sleep lose their discriminative properties to do so, treatment must then focus on altering these conditions so that they can regain their associative control with sleep. In the remainder of this chapter, each behavioral procedure and its rationale are described, and practical problems encountered in clinical practice are addressed. Sleep restriction and stimulus control procedures are summarized in Table 8.1, which is given to patients as a handout. Following is an example of how this treatment component is typically introduced to patients.

"As we discussed earlier, this intervention is divided into three main components: behavioral, cognitive, and educational. The behavioral module is further divided into two subcomponents. The first part (temporal) seeks to regulate your bedtime and arising time and to consolidate your sleep into a shorter period of time spent in bed. Insomniacs often sleep late in the morning, take daytime naps, or simply spend excessive amounts of time in bed to compensate for disturbed sleep. Accordingly, this treatment component requires that you curtail the amount of time spent in bed and that you maintain a consistent and regular sleep–wake rhythm. This objective will be achieved by strict adherence to procedures 1, 4, and 6 in the handout.

"The second part (environmental) is aimed at curtailing sleep-interfering activities that serve as cues for staying awake rather than inducing sleep. The main objective is to associate the bed, bedtime, and bedroom surroundings with relaxation, drowsiness, and sleep rather than with frustration, arousal, and sleeplessness. Accordingly, the bedroom environment should be reserved for sleep and sex only. Just as some people come to associate a certain location with better concentration or relaxation, this

**TABLE 8.1.** Sleep Restriction and Stimulus Control Procedures

---

1. Restrict the amount of time you spend in bed to the actual amount of time you sleep (i.e., ____ hours).

2. Go to bed only when you are sleepy.

3. Get out of bed if you can't fall asleep or go back to sleep within 10–15 minutes; return to bed only when you feel sleepy. Repeat this step as often as necessary during the night.

4. Maintain a regular arising time in the morning.

5. Use the bed/bedroom for sleep and sex only; do not watch TV, listen to the radio, eat, or read in bed.

6. Do not nap during the day.

---

treatment is designed to re-establish a similar association between sleep and your bed. This objective will be achieved by following procedures 2, 3, and 5 in the handout."

## Sleep Restriction

Sleep restriction consists essentially of curtailing the amount of time spent in bed (bringing it initially as close as possible to the estimated sleep time), and then gradually increasing it until an optimal sleep duration is achieved. Originally designed by Arthur Spielman (Glovinsky & Spielman, 1991; Spielman, Saskin, & Thorpy, 1987), this treatment is based on the observation that insomniacs tend to spend excessive amounts of time in bed to compensate for sleep loss and to ensure that they obtain their "required" share of sleep. Although their total sleep time does not vary a great deal from that of good sleepers, insomniacs spend substantially more time in bed to achieve the same sleep duration; their sleep efficiency is correspondingly diminished. They may go to bed early simply to ensure that they will be asleep by the desired time, stay in bed late in the morning, or take routine naps during the day. Bed rest is one of the most universal strategies to cope with temporary insomnia. It is often clinically recommended and does indeed provide some relief in the short term; however, too much time spent in bed may also yield undesirable effects, and in the long run this coping strategy is ineffective and only perpetuates insomnia. Sleep restriction is designed to circumvent these difficulties.

The following case example illustrates how to implement this procedure. Donna is a 47-year-old female who presents with a 10-year history of mixed sleep-onset and sleep-maintenance insomnia. According to her daily sleep diaries kept for a 2-week baseline period, her usual bedtime is 10:30 P.M. and she typically arises around 6:30 A.M., for a nightly mean of 8 hours spent in bed. She takes an average of 60 minutes to fall asleep and is awake for 30 minutes in the middle of the night and for an additional 30 minutes at the end of the sleep period before getting out of bed. The summation of these three variables (i.e., sleep-onset latency, wake after sleep onset, and early-morning awakening) yields a total wake time of 2 hours, leaving only 6 hours of sleep out of 8 spent in bed, for a global sleep efficiency of 75%. As described in Chapter 5, the sleep efficiency ratio (SE) is computed according to the following formula:

$$\frac{\text{Total sleep time (TST)}}{\text{Total time in bed (TIB)}} \times 100 = \text{SE}$$

Sleep restriction consists of curtailing the amount of time spent in bed to the actual or estimated amount of sleep. In this example, Donna reports sleeping an average of 6 hours per night out of 8 hours spent in bed, so the initial prescribed "sleep window" (i.e., from bedtime to arising time) is 6 hours. Allowable time in bed is subsequently adjusted contingent upon sleep efficiency. It is increased by 15–20 minutes when sleep efficiency is greater than 85% for the previous week, decreased by the same amount of time when sleep efficiency is below 80%, and kept constant when sleep efficiency falls between 80% and 85%. Periodic adjustments are made until an optimal sleep duration is reached. Ideally, the initial "sleep window" and subsequent changes in allowable time in bed are determined in an empirical fashion and according to sleep diary data. In clinical practice, however, it is not always possible or desirable to follow these rules in a rigid fashion. Adjustments are often required as a function of patients' acceptance and willingness to comply with the prescribed regimen. The following guidelines can be used in implementing sleep restriction.

1. Time in bed should rarely be restricted to less than 4–5 hours per night, no matter how poor sleep efficiency is. Further restrictions may raise strong resistance in some patients and result in noncompliance. As a general rule, it is best to initially restrict time in bed as much as the patient can tolerate. This produces a quick reversal of sleeplessness into sleepiness.

2. The specific sleep efficiency criteria used to modify allowable time in bed can also be altered according to each clinical situation. For example, my colleagues and I use slightly less stringent criteria than those originally set by Spielman, which were that time in bed was increased by 15 minutes when sleep efficiency was greater than 90% and decreased by the same amount of time when sleep efficiency was less than 85%. An alternative method is to increase time in bed contingent upon passage of time alone. After its initial curtailment, time in bed is gradually increased regardless of whether sleep efficiency reached a predetermined criterion for the previous week. Preliminary research assessing the relative efficacy of sleep restriction under time

versus sleep efficiency contingencies suggests that both methods are equally effective (Rubinstein et al., 1990). We have found this alternative quite acceptable, provided that time in bed is substantially reduced in the initial phase of the intervention (e.g., 4 or 5 hours). As treatment unfolds, however, it is preferable to resume the sleep efficiency contingency in order to prevent a return to the old habit of spending too much time awake in bed.

3. Changes in allowable time in bed are usually made on a weekly basis. It may occasionally be necessary to make more frequent changes when a patient expresses excessive concerns over sleep loss. Spielman recommends modification of the sleep schedule on a daily basis according to the sleep efficiency of the preceding five days. Such frequent alterations can be time-consuming, and for practical reasons, we prefer to make changes on a weekly basis. Regardless of the time frame adopted, any modification in time in bed should be determined prospectively by the therapist and patient. If changes are anticipated between therapy sessions, a phone call may be necessary to discuss its appropriateness.

4. Sleep restriction involves prescribing a specific "sleep window" (i.e., from bedtime to arising time), rather than a mandatory amount of time that must be spent in bed. This distinction is particularly important as stimulus control is introduced. For example, even though a patient is allowed 6 hours per night in bed, the actual time in bed may be less if the patient has to comply with the stimulus control instruction of getting out of bed when unable to fall asleep within 20 minutes (see procedure 3 in Table 8.1).

5. The patient should have control over selecting either his or her bedtime or arising time. For example, if the "sleep window" is set at 5 hours per night, the patient may choose to go to bed at 11:00 P.M., 12:00 midnight, or 1:00 A.M. However, he or she should be reminded that this schedule will require getting up 5 hours later (i.e., 4:00, 5:00, or 6:00 A.M.). To maintain consistency with stimulus control, it is preferable to keep a regular arising time and only alter the time of retiring.

6. The lower and upper limits of allowable time in bed should be based on both nighttime sleep and daytime functioning. A common side effect in the early stage of treatment is daytime sleepiness. It is important to reassure the patient that this problem is normal and only temporary. Furthermore, he or she should be reminded, "Always think of this procedure one week at a time. Do not worry as to whether you will be able to go on forever with so little sleep." Occasionally, performance and alertness can be significantly impaired to cause safety problems in people with hazardous occupations. For example, if the patient is a truck driver and complains of daytime sleepiness as a result of sleep restriction, allowable time in bed should be adjusted accordingly. Clinical judgment should guide implementation of this procedure with individuals who must drive motor vehicles or those whose jobs are potentially dangerous to themselves or others.

Sleep restriction is usually introduced to the patient in the following manner. (The actual data from the patient described above, Donna, are used here for illustrative purposes.)

"Restrict the time you spend in bed to the actual amount of sleep you get. Since you average only 6 hours of sleep per night out of 8 hours spent in bed, your task consists of curtailing the time you spend in bed to these 6 hours. There is no reason for staying in bed any longer than that, since the remaining time is spent awake anyway. Spending excessive amounts of time lying down attempting to relax, rest, nap, or simply find a comfortable body position fragments rather than consolidates sleep. Although it may have been a useful coping strategy early on, it is most likely contributing to maintaining the sleep problem currently. As your sleep becomes more efficient, you will gradually be allowed to spend more time in bed."

Sleep restriction is a somewhat paradoxical treatment for insomnia, and there is often an element of surprise when this procedure is first introduced. Some patients become concerned or anxious over the idea of drastically decreasing their time in bed, especially when their usual practice has been quite the opposite. Others are very receptive and see it as a challenge to stay awake until a predetermined time. It is often this cognitive contrast or paradox of trying to stay awake when one has been trying to fall asleep for so long that removes performance anxiety. This shift of attentional focus appears to be an important process variable that mediates sleep improvements; its effects are analogous to those achieved by paradoxical intention (Ascher & Turner, 1979).

The main effect of this procedure is to produce a mild state of sleep deprivation, which in turn produces faster sleep onset, improved sleep continuity, and a deeper sleep (more time in stages 3–4). Sleep duration is not necessarily increased, though its efficiency and quality are. Recent studies indicate that sleep restriction is a very effective intervention for insomnias of various etiologies (Friedman et al., 1991; Glovinsky & Spielman, 1991; Morin et al., 1990; Rubinstein et al., 1990; Spielman, Saskin, & Thorpy, 1987). Specific outcome results are reviewed in Chapter 12. Because sleep restriction and stimulus control procedures complement each other nicely, these two interventions are integrated in the current protocol.

## Stimulus Control

Stimulus control treatment is based on the assumption that insomnia is the result of maladaptive conditioning between environmental (bed/bedroom) and temporal (bedtime) stimuli and sleep-incompatible behaviors (e.g., worrying, reading, or watching TV in bed). According to this paradigm (Bootzin, 1972; Bootzin & Nicassio, 1978), these stimuli (bed, bedtime, and bedroom) have lost their discriminative properties previously associated with sleep. The main therapeutic goal is to re-establish or strengthen the associations between sleep and the stimulus conditions under which it typically occurs. This is accomplished by minimizing the amount of time awake in bed, by eliminating sleep-interfering activities, and by regulating the sleep–wake schedule. The basic principles operating here are analogous to those implicated with other clinical dysfunctions (e.g., obesity, substance abuse), in that the objective is to alter the relationship between a particular behavior (in this case, sleep) and the stimulus conditions (bed, bedtime, bedroom) controlling it. Bootzin has developed a set of stimulus control instructions, most recently described in Bootzin et al. (1991), that are specifically designed for insomnia. The first of these instructions (procedure 2 in Table 8.1) can be given to the patient as follows:

"Lie down intending to go to sleep only when you are drowsy. There is no reason for going to bed if you are not sleepy. When you go to bed too early, it only gives you more time to ponder events of the day, plan the schedule of tomorrow, and worry about your inability to fall asleep. Internal monologues such as these are obviously incompatible with relaxation and sleep, and tend to strengthen the negative associations between the bedroom surroundings and sleeplessness. You should therefore postpone or delay your bedtime until you are sleepy."

Insomniacs often start thinking "bedtime" right after dinnertime. To increase the likelihood of being asleep by the desired time (e.g., 11:00 P.M.), some may go to bed as early as 9:00 P.M. Although they may be tired, they are typically not sleepy by that time. So they read, watch TV, listen to music, or simply rest in bed, hoping that these activities will be sleep-inducing. Unfortunately, excessive time awake in bed heightens arousal and exacerbates sleep difficulties. Also, repeatedly engaging in these activities at bedtime means that the bed and bedroom surroundings become cues for wakefulness rather than for sleepiness.

When stimulus control therapy is being used alone, the patient's subjective level of sleepiness should determine the most appropriate bedtime. Fatigue should not be confused with true sleepiness, as this may lead to a premature bedtime and ensuing difficulties in initiating sleep. The Stanford Sleepiness Scale (Hoddes, Zarcone, Smythe, Phillips, & Dement, 1973), a 7-point Likert scale (1 = "feeling alert; wide awake," 7 = "sleep onset soon; lost struggle to remain awake"), can be used for this purpose, with the contingency that the patient will only go to bed when subjective sleepiness reaches a predetermined level. When stimulus control is combined with sleep restriction, a double standard is applied: The patient has to postpone bedtime until he or she feels sleepy, but even then the guidelines regarding the prescribed sleep window must be followed. Accordingly, if the prescribed bedtime is midnight, the patient cannot go to bed prior to that time, even though sleep is imminent by 11:00 P.M. Paradoxically, the patient may need to fight sleepiness in order to comply with the prescribed sleep window, which is exactly why the combination of these two procedures works so well.

Bedtime postponement may sometimes backfire, however. A person may be very sleepy at 11:00 P.M. but become wide awake at the prescribed bedtime of midnight. This is usually a temporary problem, which may help a person to recognize his or her true sleepiness level. The next instruction (procedure 3 in Table 8.1) is particularly useful for correcting problems associated with a premature bedtime:

"If you are unable to fall asleep or return to sleep within 10–15 minutes, get out of bed, go into another room, and engage in some quiet activity. You can read, listen to music, watch a pretaped movie, or practice any similar nonstimulating activities. Do not sleep on the couch. Return to bed only when sleepy. Repeat this step as often as necessary throughout the night—that is, when you first go to bed and upon nocturnal awakening. It will be difficult and demanding to follow this instruction. However, consistent adherence to this regimen will help reassociate your bed/bedroom with getting to sleep *quickly*."

For many patients, this is one of the most difficult instructions to comply with. Poor sleepers typically toss and turn and repeatedly postpone their getting out of bed. The underlying belief is that if they keep trying, sleep will eventually come. If nothing else, most of them prefer to stay in bed, assuming that at least they are getting some rest. It is more detrimental to toss and turn and worry about falling asleep than actually to get out of bed and do something else until sleep is imminent. An excessive amount of time awake in bed exacerbates both performance anxiety and insomnia. Diligent adherence to this procedure is essential to break the vicious cycle of insomnia, arousal, and further sleep disturbances. There is no need for the patient to watch the clock constantly, as this alone will heighten arousal and worsen sleep difficulties, but the clinician should clearly emphasize the need to follow this instruction as consistently as possible. A similar emphasis is necessary with the next instruction (procedure 4 in Table 8.1):

"Maintain a regular arising time. Set the alarm clock and get out of bed at approximately the same time every morning, weekdays and weekends, regardless of your bedtime or the amount of sleep obtained on the previous night. Although it may be tempting to stay in bed later because you haven't slept well on the previous night, try to maintain a steady sleep schedule. It helps regulate your internal biological clock and synchronize your sleep–wake rhythm."

This procedure may need to be slightly altered when used in conjunction with sleep restriction. Ideally, only bedtime changes when the sleep window is modified. During the early phase of treatment, however, the arising time may need to be altered as well, depending on a patient's preference. Arising times that stay within a 2-hour range (5:30–7:30 A.M.) are acceptable.

The next stimulus control instruction (procedure 5 in Table 8.1) can be presented as follows:

"Use the bed or bedroom for sleep only. Do not read, eat, watch TV, work, or worry in your bed/bedroom either during the day or at night. Sex is the only exception to this rule. When you engage in these practices in your bedroom, this environment becomes associated with wakefulness rather than with sleepiness. Curtailing nonsleeping activities in the bedroom will reinforce the associations between that environment and sleep. Just as you may have developed strong associations between the kitchen and hunger or between a particular chair and relaxation, the main objective here is to re-establish a strong association between sleep and the bedroom surroundings."

For many people, the bedroom is the center of their universe. They tend to organize their entire daily activities within that surrounding. Eating, reading, watching TV, paying the bills, and talking on the phone are just a few examples of these sleep-incompatible activities. Because of physical discomfort and restricted range of motions, some older adults and patients with chronic medical illnesses are particularly likely to engage in these practices (Morin & Gramling, 1990; Morin, Kowatch, & Wade, 1989). Some couples use the bedroom or bedtime as a place and time to problem-solve marital, sexual, or child-rearing difficulties. The main objective of this instruction is to strengthen the cueing properties of the bedroom environment for sleep. This procedure is theoretically supported by the extensive literature on classical conditioning and more specifically by that on stimulus discrimination. Although some individuals who engage in sleep-incompatible behaviors do not necessarily have trouble sleeping, others may be more susceptible to these underlying conditioning processes. Those who are more prone to insomnia and who display these maladaptive behaviors should simply eliminate these practices altogether. Although many patients initially report not engaging in these activities, the clinician may find out after repeated inquiries that they do indeed watch TV, problem-solve on the pillow, and occasionally have a snack or read in bed. Individuals living in one-room apartments should use a divider between the bed and the rest of the room.

The final stimulus control instruction (procedure 6 in Table 8.1) can be introduced in this manner:

"It is best to avoid daytime napping. When you stay awake all day, you are more sleepy at night. Routine daytime napping disrupts the natural sleep–wake rhythm and interferes with nighttime sleep. However, if daytime sleepiness is too overwhelming, a short nap not to exceed 1 hour and scheduled before 3:00 P.M. is permissible."

Routine daytime napping usually interferes with nighttime sleep. The speed of sleep onset is inversely related to the length of the previous episode of wakefulness (Webb & Agnew, 1975). The longer the wake period, the shorter the latency to sleep onset. In addition, a late afternoon or evening nap is more detrimental to the following night's sleep than a morning nap. Research on circadian rhythms shows that slow-wave sleep is concentrated in the early part of the night, whereas REM sleep is more predominant in the second half. Accordingly, a late afternoon or evening nap is made up of more slow-wave sleep, which is borrowed from the upcoming night's sleep, whereas the earlier nap is more like a continuation of the previous sleep episode.

Specific advice on daytime napping may vary according to the patient population and the phase of treatment. Routine daytime napping is usually discouraged, particularly in younger patients. There are a few instances, however, in which it may be permissible. First, in the early phase of sleep restriction, a limited nap is made optional when there is an excessive concern about restricting time in bed. Also, when daytime sleepiness is overwhelming, a short nap may be recommended to people who have to drive motor vehicles or perform hazardous occupations. As treatment unfolds and nocturnal time in bed is increased, this option is gradually phased out. Second, because it seems to interfere less with the night sleep of older adults (Aber & Webb, 1986), napping is also optional in the management of late-life insomnia. Third, some insomniacs apparently sleep better at night after a daytime nap. For those few exceptions, napping should be limited to no more than 1 hour and scheduled before 3:00 P.M., as stated above, in order to minimize interference with nighttime sleep. To strenghten the discriminative properties of the bedroom environment for sleep, napping should be done at a regular time and in bed. It should also be curtailed if no sleep has occurred within 15–20 minutes of getting into bed.

A final procedure that the therapist may introduce at this point is not among Bootzin's stimulus control instructions (or included in Table 8.1), but it may be an important one for some patients:

"Allow yourself at least an hour before bedtime to unwind. Use this transitional period to engage in your prebedtime rituals (reading, bathing, brushing teeth, etc.). Do not rehash events of the day or plan tomorrow's schedule. Set aside another time during the day or early evening to do problem solving and to write down worries or concerns."

Although this last procedure is not part of the standard stimulus control format, it is often essential to remind patients to prepare themselves for sleep in the same manner they would prepare for a journey. Some people work until the very last minute before getting into bed; failure to allow for a transitional period is likely to result in excessive cognitive arousal, which will naturally delay the onset of sleep.

Several comparative studies have shown that stimulus control is the treatment of choice for disorders of initiating sleep (Espie, Lindsay, Brooks, et al., 1989; Lacks, Bertelson, Gans, & Kunkel, 1983; Ladouceur & Gros-Louis, 1986; Turner & Ascher, 1979) and maintaining sleep (Lacks, Bertelson, Sugerman, & Kunkel, 1983; Morin & Azrin, 1987, 1988; Schoicket et al., 1988). Component analyses assessing the relative efficacy of temporal and environmental instructions have found no difference between procedures aimed at regulating sleep schedules (temporal) and those aimed at curtailing sleep-incompatible behaviors (environmental). Combined instruction sets proved superior to either component alone (Tokartz & Lawrence, 1974; Zwart & Lisman, 1979).

## Enhancing Treatment Credibility and the Patient's Adherence

Once the various procedures and their rationale have been described, the therapist may provide additional background information about their developmental history and clinical effectiveness. This information is useful to enhance treatment credibility, to induce a sense of hope in those patients who thought their insomnia was hopeless, and to caution others against excessive optimism.

"These procedures have been developed by clinical psychologists as an alternative to more traditional therapies and drug treatments. They have been extensively tested in several clinics throughout the world and have been shown to be effective with other patients suffering similar insomnia problems. About 75% of chronic insomniacs benefit from this intervention, with an average improvement rate of 50–60% in the reduction of sleep-onset latency and/or time awake after sleep onset. Although it is no miracle cure for all insomnia problems, this treatment will help you develop self-management skills and regain control of sleep, so you can cope with occasional sleep difficulties that you may encounter even after completing this program."

To foster treatment adherence, it is important to relate each procedure to the patient's goals and to point out its clinical relevance in light of the maladaptive sleep habits that have perpetuated insomnia. A detailed history and a careful functional analysis of the sleep problem during the initial evaluation will facilitate this task.

"This intervention is a highly structured regimen that requires time, patience, and effort. To achieve your goals of falling asleep quickly at bedtime and of reducing the time spent awake in the middle of the night, it is important that you comply with all procedures. You cannot choose only those that seem least painful. You may find that sleep gets worse the first few nights of practice and that you wake up in the morning feeling more exhausted than usual. Do not get discouraged, as this is normal early in treatment. Benefits will become more evident with time and repeated practice. The most important factor determining whether sleep will improve or not is the consistency with which you follow the various instructions. Individuals who comply carefully with our recommendations usually start noticing marked improvement in their sleep patterns after 6–8 weeks of practice."

## Clinical Issues and Problems

The clinical procedures reviewed so far are fairly straightforward, at least on paper. Nevertheless, several problems are likely to arise during the course of their implementation. Some of these problems stem directly from patients' noncompliance; others are the result of clinicians' misconceptions about the management of insomnia. The behavioral treatment component is primarily didactic in nature and does not involve rehearsal or training during the therapy sessions, as would be required with relaxation training, for example. A common ensuing mistake made by some clinicians is to assume that their job is over once the procedures have been described. Clearly, simply handing out a behavioral prescription without proper follow-up will almost inevitably lead to treatment failure. Much clinical work remains to be done in subsequent sessions. The therapist's role is (1) to ensure that patients understand the procedures and their rationale; and (2) to foster strict adherence with the prescribed regimen through constant support, direct guidance, and problem solving of difficulties encountered during home practice. Before problems of noncompliance are addressed, general issues concerned with treatment implementation and objections commonly raised by patients are reviewed.

Should these procedures be implemented all at once or in a stepwise fashion? Our usual practice is to introduce all procedures together and implement them in a gradual fashion. Patients' acceptance and willingness to comply with the proposed regimen may dictate the most appropriate method to follow. When a patient is anxious about decreasing his or her time in bed, it is preferable to begin with the stimulus control instructions only. Conversely, those who are resistant to getting out of bed if they are unable to fall asleep may be more receptive to sleep restriction. In the early phase of treatment, the initial reduction of time in bed may override the need for using some of the stimulus control instructions. For instance, if the sleep window is substantially restricted, the sleep drive will be strong enough at bedtime that it will almost override the need to get out of bed. As time in bed is increased, the need to use these instructions will be greater.

A frequent issue raised by some patients is that they do not engage in sleep-incompatible behaviors, do not nap, and do not sleep late in the morning. It is indeed quite possible that not all procedures are equally relevant for a given patient. In most cases, however, specific maladaptive behaviors that are instrumental in perpetuating sleep difficulties can always be uncovered by refining the initial functional analysis and by having the patient engage in additional self-monitoring of sleep patterns. Furthermore, sleep restriction will always be clinically relevant, provided that significant difficulties in initiating or maintaining sleep are present.

Sleep is a topic of popular interest that receives a great deal of media coverage. Prior exposure to some of the clinical procedures outlined in this program is not unusual. Some patients may claim that they have tried implementing these techniques on their own but failed to notice changes in their sleep patterns. Treatment integrity, or the lack thereof, is unfortunately a common problem in any self-management program. The clinician should, first, reinforce the fact that a patient is knowledgeable about self-management techniques, and second, point out specific obstacles that may have impeded previous efforts. The absolute need for consistent adherence to the entire regimen over a sufficiently long period of time should be re-emphasized. The clinician may also point out that he or she will provide direct guidance and ongoing corrective feedback to counter problems that may have been overlooked in the past. After that, it is a matter of obtaining a firm commitment from patients to follow through on these recommendations and give this program another trial.

## Strategies for Overcoming Difficulties with Treatment Adherence

### Difficulties in Postponing Bedtime

Patients may raise several objections to postponing bedtime. The fear of missing the most refreshing portion of a night's sleep and, paradoxically, the inability to stay awake until the prescribed bedtime are the two most common ones. In the first scenario, the popular belief that the best sleep is obtained before midnight can be altered by pointing out that deep sleep, though predominant in the first third of the night, will always occur first (within some limits) regardless of one's bedtime. When the sleep period is curtailed, it is usually REM sleep—which is more predominant in the last third of the night—that is diminished. Cognitive therapy will focus more directly on altering this dysfunctional belief. To counter the second objection (i.e., inability to stay awake until the prescribed bedtime), a list of competing activities should be generated to fight sleepiness. These are typically physical (e.g., household work, needlework) rather than cognitive (e.g., reading) or passive (e.g., watching TV) in nature. It may also include having someone come over to visit in the evening, talking on the phone with a friend, or any similar activities that are incompatible with sleep. Obviously, some of these activities may not be realistic if bedtime is postponed too late in the night.

## Failure to Get Out of Bed When Unable to Fall Asleep

In examining the patient's sleep diary for a given week, if sleep latencies exceed 20–30 minutes for any given night, the therapist should first inquire whether the patient got out of bed on those occasions. Failure to do so is one of the problems most frequently encountered with stimulus control therapy. It is necessary to inquire about potential factors preventing adherence to this advice. "I'm afraid it's going to wake me up even more," "It's too cold," "I don't know what to do," or "I'm afraid of waking up my bed partner" are the most common objections. Because these are legitimate concerns, the therapist needs to use convincing arguments to promote adherence to this instruction.

First, the rationale for getting out of bed should be reiterated. It should not be presented as a punishment, but rather as a means of reassociating the bed with falling asleep quickly. It may be necessary to explain over and over again that the practice of lying in bed awake trying harder to go to sleep only increases anxiety, frustration, and further sleep disturbances. Only getting out of bed can short-circuit this vicious cycle. Second, each objection needs to be addressed and a solution designed accordingly. Some recommendations include leaving a blanket on the couch if it is too cold in the winter months, or planning ahead of time nonstimulating activities for the middle of the night. It is also important to inquire whether the bed partner has ever complained of being awakened. Usually he or she is deeply asleep and doesn't notice the patient's getting up. However, if this is indeed a problem, the therapist might consider asking the patient to move to a different bedroom for the duration of treatment.

## Waiting Too Long before Getting Out of Bed

Some patients may get out of bed, but simply wait too long before doing so, thereby defeating the purpose of this instruction. Every time they think of getting out of bed, they also believe that sleep is imminent and postpone their getting up. A good rule of thumb to foster compliance with this instruction is to make the time out of bed contingent upon the time spent in bed prior to getting up. For example, if a patient waits 25 minutes before getting out of bed, he or she should plan on staying up for at least the same duration.

This rule serves as an incentive not to exceed the prescribed limits of 15–20 minutes in bed before getting up. Once again, although a patient should not constantly watch the clock, staying in bed awake too long will impede treatment progress.

## Returning to Bed Too Quickly

A common mistake in implementing the "get out of bed" instruction is to return to bed too quickly. Often patients just pace the floor for a few minutes and are eager to return to bed, fearing that if they stay up too long, they will never go back to sleep. To alleviate this apprehension, it is important to point out that the longer the patients stay up, the quicker they will fall asleep when they return to bed, provided that they stop worrying about the next-day deficits. Some patients fail to recognize their true sleepiness level. Just as there are large discrepancies between subjective and objective sleep parameters, subjective and objective sleepiness levels are also quite divergent. It is helpful to identify behavioral cues of sleepiness (e.g., yawning, heavy eyelids) for selecting the most appropriate time for returning to bed. Use of the Stanford Sleepiness Scale or any similar scale may also prove useful for this purpose.

## Oversleeping in the Morning

Catching up on sleep over the weekends is a fairly common practice to prevent chronic sleep deprivation. Insomnia sufferers, however, are particularly vulnerable to the negative consequences of such practices. Oversleeping on weekends disrupts natural circadian rhythms and only leads to more severe insomnia on Sunday nights. Adherence to a strict and regular arising time is likely to become problematic, particularly as the sleep restriction procedure is implemented. Sleep deprivation deepens subsequent sleep and also raises the awakening threshold. Getting out of bed for extended periods makes it more difficult to arise at the prescribed time. The first step to deal with this problem is to make sure that an alarm clock is used even by those who report waking up before their desired arising time. Second, scheduling social activities or family commitments may increase motivation for getting out of bed early on weekends. A bed partner can be instrumental in encouraging a patient to comply with this instruction, though this responsibility should ultimately be assumed by the patient alone. Third, a leeway of a couple of hours in arising times may be more acceptable, especially in younger patients, and should not defeat the purpose of this procedure.

## Falling Asleep in Places Other than the Bedroom

Poor sleepers usually fall asleep more easily when they are not trying (e.g., reading, watching TV) and in a nonsleeping environment (e.g., on the couch or in a reclining chair). These practices should be discouraged during the course of treatment, in order to strengthen the bed/bedroom as the main discriminative stimulus for sleep. A spouse or partner can be helpful in minimizing the occurrence of such practices.

## Reading in Bed as a Sleep-Inducing Technique

Reading or watching TV in bed around bedtime is sleep-inducing for some people. Not surprisingly, insomniacs are reluctant to give up such practices, which have become part of their bedtime routines. Several issues should be considered when addressing this problem. First, how long does it take to fall asleep after getting into bed and reading or watching TV? If sleep-onset latency is 1 or 2 hours, these activities are clearly not sleep-inducing. On the other hand, if sleep comes within 30 minutes of getting to bed, then there is probably no significant problem with initiating sleep. Second, is it the patient or the bed partner who enjoys this prebedtime ritual? In the latter case, it may be necessary for the patient to negotiate with the bed partner for the removal of a TV from the bedroom. Third, is the bedroom the only quiet and private place where the patient can engage in these activities? An alternate quiet and private room should be identified to practice these activities during the day or at bedtime.

I have reviewed the most common difficulties encountered in implementing the behavioral treatment component. This is clearly not an exhaustive list of problems, but instead a sampling of the most common ones to expect and be prepared for. Some of these problems will be more easily addressed when the cognitive therapy component is introduced.

## Conclusion

A number of behavioral practices are helpful in coping with the debilitating effects of acute insomnia. These same practices, however, are often instrumental in exacerbating and perpetuating the initial sleep problem. Regardless of the specific triggering factors that initially precipitated the insomnia, direct alteration of the current maladaptive behavior patterns is an essential element for the effective management of chronic insomnia. Of all psychological interventions, stimulus control and sleep restriction are the two most effective treatment modalities for sleep-onset and sleep-maintenance insomnia (Lacks & Morin, 1992). Their effectiveness, either alone or in combination, has been documented with healthy young adults (Espie, Lindsay, Brooks, et al., 1989; Lacks, Bertelson, Gans, & Kunkel, 1983; Lacks, Bertelson, Sugerman, & Kunkel, 1983; Spielman, Sasky, & Thorpy, 1987; Turner & Ascher, 1979), with middle-aged and older people (Edinger, Hoelscher, Marsh, Lipper, & Ionescu-Pioggia, 1992; Engle-Friedman, Bootzin, Hazlewood, & Tsao, 1992; Friedman et al., 1991; Hoelscher & Edinger, 1988; Morin & Azrin, 1987, 1988; Morin, Kowatch, et al., 1993), with chronic pain patients (Morin, Kowatch, & Wade, 1989), and even with inpatients (Edinger, Lipper, & Wheeler, 1989; Morin et al., 1990).

# 9

# Cognitive Therapy Component

Cognitive therapy has received little attention in the management of insomnia, relative to the management of other psychological disorders. Clinical and research efforts have predominantly focused on modifying overt maladaptive behaviors, with little emphasis placed on the beliefs and attitudes underlying insomnia. Faulty appraisal, unrealistic expectations, and misattributions of the causes and consequences of insomnia are particularly relevant targets for intervention. In this chapter I outline several dysfunctional sleep cognitions and illustrate their effective alteration with cognitive restructuring techniques. These procedures have been modeled after the work of Aaron Beck, Albert Ellis, and Donald Meichenbaum and adapted to insomnia problems.

## The Role of Cognitive Factors in Insomnia

As described in more detail in Chapter 4, psychological research on insomnia etiology has predominantly focused on contrasting the relative influence of cognitive and physiological arousal (Gross & Borkovec, 1982; Freedman & Sattler, 1982; Haynes et al., 1981; Lichstein & Rosenthal, 1980). Although cognitive arousal in the form of excessive mentation or intrusive thoughts is more strongly associated with sleep disruptions than is somatic arousal, it is still unclear whether it causes insomnia or simply represents an epiphenomenon of nighttime wakefulness. Several authors have emphasized the importance of emotional arousal as a potential mediating factor (Lacks, 1987; Espie, 1991). There is also an increasing amount of evidence suggesting that the content and affective tone of sleep-related cognitions play a greater role than the rate of cognitive activity alone in mediating insomnia. For example, insomniacs tend to endorse state (presleep) and trait (daytime) measures reflecting an anxious, dysphoric, and worrisome cognitive style (Borkovec et al., 1981; Edinger et al., 1988; A. Kales & Kales, 1984; Van Egeren et al., 1983), and these features correlate with sleep difficulties. In addition, insomniacs hold more unrealistic expectations about their sleep requirements, stronger beliefs about the negative consequences of insomnia, and more external and unstable causal attributions of their sleep difficulties than normal controls. These dysfunctional cognitions are associated with both emotional distress and sleep disturbances (Morin et al., in press; Van Egeren et al., 1983).

Collectively, this evidence suggests that maladaptive cognitions are instrumental in producing emotional arousal, which in turn perpetuates insomnia. Accordingly, the cognitive therapy module focuses on altering these cognitions. It does not rely on methods that directly attempt to control excessive ruminations (e.g., imagery training, thought stopping). Rather, the focus is on altering the underlying dysfunctional thinking processes and affective responses through cognitive restructuring procedures. I now review several of these concepts and discuss their interrelationships with insomnia.

1. *Faulty appraisal* of transient sleep difficulties is a common triggering point of chronic insomnia. Disturbed sleep is more likely to be distressing when it is perceived as reflecting a loss of personal control than when it is evaluated in terms of extenuating circumstances. For example, viewing a poor night's sleep as the result of a hectic day at work or family conflicts at home is more adaptive than interpreting it as evidence of losing control over the ability to sleep. The latter interpretation may lead to performance anxiety and learned helplessness, and thus may aggravate the sleep problem.

2. *Misattributions* of daytime impairments to poor sleep can feed into this self-fulfilling prophecy. Sleep is an easy target, and insomniacs have a tendency to blame it for everything that goes wrong during the day. Fatigue, lowered energy, performance decrements, and mood disturbances are often attributed to poor sleep. Some of these sequelae may indeed result from disturbed sleep, but the exclusive attribution of all daytime misfortunes to insomnia is counterproductive. A variety of alternative factors, such as natural circadian changes, stress in other areas of life, and a poor coping style in general, can cause these impairments.

3. *Unrealistic expectations* regarding sleep requirements are equally important. Although most people rarely think about how much sleep they need, insomniacs tend to hold stronger and more definite beliefs about their own needs. For example, the belief that 8 hours of sleep is essential to maintain adequate daytime functioning is common among poor sleepers. Self-imposing such a rigid standard, however, only increases performance anxiety and interferes with the process of falling asleep. Unfortunately, sleep does not come on command. It is a natural process that can only be facilitated by lowering physiological, emotional, and cognitive arousal.

4. Several types of cognitive errors are involved in the vicious cycle of insomnia, emotional distress, and more sleep disturbances. *Excessive ruminations, magnification, catastrophizing, overgeneralization, dichotomous think-*

*ing, and selective recall* contribute to this self-perpetuating system in the very same fashion as they do to other psychological dysfunctions (Beck et al., 1979; Beck, Emery, & Greenberg, 1985; Freeman, Pretzer, Fleming, & Simon, 1990; Meichenbaum, 1985; Turk, Meichenbaum, & Genest, 1983).

Perceptual distortions are fairly common among insomnia sufferers. There is a tendency to magnify the intensity of sleep difficulties, as well as the resulting daytime sequelae. Dwelling on sleep loss and worrying about its presumed consequences only aggravate insomnia problems. Although performance decrements that can be specifically attributed to disturbed sleep are limited, excessive concerns about those presumed consequences make matters worse by increasing anxiety and lowering tolerance for temporary sleep loss. Excessive worrying sometimes turns into catastrophizing. After several consecutive sleepless nights, it is not uncommon for insomniacs to reach a state of panic. Some question whether they will ever be able to go to sleep again, and others believe they may have a nervous breakdown if sleep does not come soon. Catastrophizing is often sparked by the personal conviction that sleeplessness is necessarily detrimental to physical and mental health. The extensive night-to-night variability in sleep patterns of insomniacs is often accompanied by a natural tendency to selectively recall only the bad nights and overlook the good ones. The sleep diary is extremely helpful in uncovering this selective focus. Overgeneralization plays a corollary role, in that insomniacs may come to their therapy session claiming that their entire week of sleep was inadequate when in fact they had two or three good nights for that particular week. Dichotomous thinking is best exemplified when patients describe their sleep in an all-or-none fashion (e.g., "awful," "restless," "miserable"). There are rarely half measures with insomnia sufferers.

5. Dysfunctional sleep cognitions are strongly intertwined with *emotional distress and maladaptive behavior patterns.* For instance, insomnia is frequently accompanied by mixed features of anxiety and depression. The direction of the relationship between sleep and mood disturbances is often unclear, but it is usually further complicated by various dysfunctional cognitions and by poor sleep habits. For example, the belief that it is essential to make up for sleep loss may lead a patient to spend excessive amounts of time in bed. In turn, spending too much time in bed exacerbates sleep difficulties, triggers further negative emotions, and reinforces the erroneous belief that control over sleep is effectively lacking.

## Treatment Goals and Rationale

The primary goal of cognitive therapy is to guide patients to re-evaluate the accuracy of their thinking about sleeplessness, its causal factors, and presumed consequences. The main issue here is not to deny the presence of sleep difficulties or their impact on daytime functioning; instead, the objective is to view insomnia from a more realistic perspective and short-circuit its self-fulfilling nature. Although some of the themes covered here have already been discussed in Chapter 8, cognitive therapy specifically targets the beliefs and attitudes giving rise to the behavior patterns described earlier. The basic premise of this approach is that dysfunctional covert processes mediate the development and perpetuation of insomnia by producing negative emotional responses and by leading patients to engage in maladaptive behavior patterns. Alterations of the underlying cognitive processes should then alleviate psychological distress, curtail bad sleep habits, and ultimately improve sleep patterns.

Although complete cure would be an ideal goal, the reality is that most patients will continue to experience occasional sleep difficulties even after undergoing the full intervention. Cognitive therapy is particularly relevant in this context, because it teaches patients strategies to cope more adaptively with these residual problems after treatment. By changing appraisal of an occasional poor night's sleep, which virtually everyone experiences at one time or another, cognitive interventions play an important role in preventing relapse into full-fledged chronic insomnia. Also, because patients often perceive themselves as victims of insomnia, an important goal of treatment is to strengthen their sense of control in coping with the sleep problem (Bootzin, 1985).

## Cognitive Therapy Procedures

The main clinical procedures used to achieve the aforementioned goals are cognitive restructuring techniques such as reappraisal, reattribution, and decatastrophizing. The patient is guided to re-examine the validity of his or her beliefs and to reframe them with more adaptive substitutes. Implementation of these procedures involves three sequential steps: (1) identifying dysfunctional sleep cognitions, (2) challenging their validity, and (3) replacing them with more adaptive substitutes. First, however, two preparatory steps are necessary.

The first one is to provide patients with a conceptual framework of the interrelationship among cognition, affect, and behavior. This process is facilitated by starting off with examples unrelated to sleep disturbances; patients are generally more receptive to such examples and can thus gain a better perspective on this interaction. We usually select hypothetical situations likely to trigger various negative emotions. The patient is asked to think of a personal situation that made him or her anxious, depressed, or angry, and to verbalize specific self-statements accompanying these emotional upsets. The therapist then proceeds to demonstrate how these same principles operate

**TABLE 9.1.** Relationships between Sleep Cognitions and Affect

| Situation | Cognitions/thoughts | Feelings |
|---|---|---|
| Eating breakfast in the morning | "How am I gonna get through the day after such a miserable night?" | Depressed, helpless |
| Poor functioning at work | "I just can't do my work after a bad night's sleep." | Angry, irritable |
| Watching TV in the evening | "I must have some sleep tonight." | Anxious or apprehensive |
| Getting ready for bed | "What's the use of going to bed tonight when I know I won't be able to go to sleep?" | Helpless, out of control |

in the context of sleep disturbances. Table 9.1, which may be given to patients as a handout, presents examples of typical self-statements made by insomniacs in various situations. Figure 4.2 is also helpful in illustrating how dysfunctional cognitions perpetuate insomnia.

The second step consists of explaining to patients the basic principles of cognitive therapy and the rationale for targeting their beliefs and attitudes. A didactic approach should be used, and the language should be adapted to each patient's educational level and psychological sophistication. Following is an example of how we typically introduce cognitive therapy to patients:

"We have thus far concentrated on changing poor sleep habits. As you make these behavioral changes part of your new lifestyle, we also need to examine your attitudes and beliefs about sleep and insomnia. The way people think about a particular problem can either alleviate or aggravate that problem. What you think also affects how you feel and what you do. For example, when you worry during the day about how poorly you slept the night before, it is likely to make you more apprehensive about the upcoming night. Excessive concerns about the consequences of poor sleep can feed into your problem as well. An overly preoccupied mind and emotional upset are not very conducive to sleep. Accordingly, this treatment component is designed to help you address these concerns. To regain greater self-control over sleep, you must first set aside previously held beliefs and replace them with more adaptive ones."

## Identifying Dysfunctional Sleep Cognitions

Uncovering dysfunctional thoughts about sleep is the first task of cognitive therapy. Some patients are often unaware of these covert events; others, convinced that insomnia is a sign of weakness, are simply unwilling to disclose their personal beliefs or self-statements. As a result, they also fail to realize how these factors influence the development of anxious or dysphoric emotions feeding into their sleep disturbances. Thus, increasing patients' awareness is an integral component of treatment.

Systematic self-monitoring is the best strategy to achieve this goal and to desensitize patients about sharing these beliefs with the therapist. Training is often essential to help patients obtain adequate records of thoughts, beliefs, and expectations, because of their automatic quality and inconspicuous nature. It is important to point out to patients that these self-statements continually flow through their minds in response to external events (e.g., a bad night's sleep, poor work performance). Although not everyone engages in this process to the same extent, virtually every insomniac entertains some thoughts about the causes and consequences of poor sleep. Insomniacs are especially prone to excessive rumination. They spend more time thinking and worrying about their personal problems and sleep difficulties than do good sleepers (Marchini et al., 1983). Their typical psychological profile is one of internalizing and worrying, leading to self-scrutiny.

As a starting point, the clinician can refer to the patient's responses on the Beliefs and Attitudes about Sleep instrument (Appendix C). This scale is useful in generating an initial list of dysfunctional cognitions. Daily self-monitoring should supplement this information, as some people may entertain different and more personally relevant cognitions. To facilitate recognition, the patient may also be asked to imagine himself or herself in situations such as the following and to report thoughts triggered by these situations.

THERAPIST: Close your eyes and listen carefully to this. It's 1:30 A.M., and you have been lying wide awake in bed since 11:30 P.M. You have been tossing and turning for the past 2 hours, but nothing seems to make you sleepy. If anything, you seem to be getting more awake. You keep thinking about this presentation you have to give tomorrow morning. Now, I would like you to tell me what goes through your mind right at this moment.

PATIENT: Well, I feel that I'm getting uptight and tense. I have to go to sleep pretty soon; otherwise I'll be a mess tomorrow. I've got 5 hours left before getting up. If I don't get to sleep soon, I know I won't be able to give a good presentation.

THERAPIST: You're at work and it's 3:00 in the afternoon. Your sleep was miserable last night. You've been trying to complete this project, but you just can't seem to concentrate and work efficiently today.

PATIENT: I get upset when I can't function any better than that. I know it's because I didn't sleep well last night. Tonight I'm going to bed early. I really need to get a good night's sleep; otherwise I know I'll be a zombie tomorrow.

This "induced imagery" technique (Beck et al., 1979) provides a better understanding of the types of self-statements a patient must be attentive to. These examples can be used for illustrative purposes in completing entries on a daily record of automatic thoughts (which can be structured like Table 9.1). Patients are then instructed to monitor samples of sleep-related thoughts that trigger negative emotions either during the day or at night.

## Exploring, Clarifying, and Challenging the Validity of Cognitions

After patient-specific self-statements are identified, their validity should be explored. Training in viewing one's explanations, interpretations, and expectations as hypotheses rather than absolute truths is the first step. Then the clinician confronts erroneous beliefs/attitudes giving rise to these schemata. To facilitate this task, my colleagues and I often make reference to recent research findings and contrast these with popular beliefs that have shaped our patients' own belief systems. A therapist must be cautious to avoid antagonizing a patient with dogmatic statements such as "Not everyone needs 8 hours of sleep" or "It's all in your mind." Rather, it is best to encourage him or her to explore alternative hypotheses and to test them by experimenting with various sleep durations, by systematically assessing their impact on daytime functioning, and by attempting to go on with the usual routines despite disturbed sleep. These homework assignments often diminish excessive concerns, shift the exclusive focus on sleeplessness, and enhance awareness that daytime functioning is not exclusively dependent upon the previous night's sleep.

## Providing More Adaptive and Rational Substitute Cognitions

The third step of cognitive restructuring consists of providing more adaptive substitutes for the patient's dysfunctional thought patterns. This is best accomplished by using techniques of reattribution, reinterpretation, reappraisal, hypothesis testing, and decatastrophizing (Beck et al., 1979, 1985; Freeman et al., 1990; Meichenbaum, 1977). Direct guidance is essential at this stage. The next section illustrates how to implement these procedures.

## Altering Beliefs and Attitudes about Sleep

Dysfunctional sleep cognitions are of five types: (1) misconceptions of the causes of insomnia, (2) misattributions or amplifications of its consequences, (3) unrealistic sleep expectations, (4) diminished perceptions of control and predictability of sleep, and (5) faulty beliefs about sleep-promoting practices. After each type is introduced, a series of vignettes illustrates its presentation in clinical practice and the underlying maladaptive information processing. Cognitive restructuring interventions designed to replace the dysfunctional cognitions with more adaptive substitutes are then outlined.

## Correcting Misconceptions of Insomnia Causes

Individuals often come to therapy with very definite explanations accounting for their insomnia. Common causal attributions include pain, allergy, menopause, age, depression, or some forms of chemical imbalance. The basic assumption underlying such explanations is that only when these physical, hormonal, developmental, or biochemical factors are addressed can the sleep problem be resolved. Although some of these attributions may be valid, they essentially remain outside a patient's reach in the present therapeutic context. Such formulations also lead the patient to adopt a passive stance vis-à-vis the problem, and self-efficacy and outcome expectations are correspondingly diminished. Common misconceptions about the causes of insomnia are illustrated in Vignettes 9.1 and 9.2.

The main objective of cognitive therapy is to alter these external and unidimensional explanations of insomnia. The patient is first trained to distinguish the origins of his or her sleep problem from the current perpetuating factors. This is most effectively accomplished by referring to Figure 4.1, which illustrates the developmental course of insomnia. Second, while the influence of precipitating factors is acknowledged, the patient is guided to reattribute some of the current causes to factors he or she has some control over. The rationale invoked here is that regardless of the nature of the

**VIGNETTE 9.1.** Misconceptions of Insomnia Causes

---

| | |
|---|---|
| *Dysfunctional Cognition:* | "I feel my insomnia is basically the result of some biochemical imbalance or pain." |
| *Underlying Belief:* | "Unless these underlying problems are corrected, there is nothing I can do to improve my sleep." |
| *Cognitive Errors:* | Misattribution, faulty evidence, absolute thinking. |

*Interventions/Alternative Interpretations:*
(1) Exclusive attribution of insomnia to these external causes is self-defeating because you may indeed have little control over them.
(2) Regardless of the initial precipitating causes, psychological and behavioral variables are almost always involved in chronic insomnia.
(3) Because you have some control in changing these variables, you can also improve your sleep patterns.

---

VIGNETTE 9.2. Other Misconceptions of Insomnia Causes

---

| | |
|---|---|
| *Dysfunctional Cognition:* | "I feel my sleep problem is essentially the result of aging and I can't do anything about it." |
| *Underlying Belief:* | "Disturbed sleep is an inevitable consequence of aging." |
| *Cognitive Errors:* | Misattribution, faulty evidence, absolute thinking. |

*Interventions/Alternative Interpretations:*
(1) Do all older people you know have sleep disturbances?
(2) Beyond some normal age-related changes in sleep patterns, not all older people suffer from insomnia; therefore, other factors must be involved.
(3) Lifestyle changes accompanying retirement may alter your sleep patterns; thus, you can make some adjustments in these areas to improve sleep.

---

precipitating factors that initially triggered the insomnia, psychological and behavioral factors are playing a key role in maintaining it over time. The underlying message conveyed is that the patient has some control over these factors. By altering their presence, he or she can learn to overcome (or at least to cope more adaptively with) disturbed sleep.

"Attributing insomnia solely to external causes, as in statements such as 'My sleep problem is entirely due to pain' or 'Because I am getting older, it is normal to have sleep problems,' is self-defeating. Although age, pain, or physical ailments may contribute to sleep difficulties, psychological factors can either alleviate or exacerbate those difficulties. Thus, it is important to adopt a more constructive attitude and assume some control over these factors."

After some of the misconceptions about the causes of insomnia are reviewed, the next step consists of exploring the other side of the coin—that is, the presumed consequences of disturbed sleep.

## Reattributing the Presumed Consequences of Insomnia

One of the most common reasons prompting insomnia sufferers to seek therapy is not so much the sleep problem itself as the fear of its presumed consequences. This fear revolves primarily around excessive concerns about the ill effects of poor sleep on performance efficiency, psychological well-being, and physical health. Although there are well-documented consequences of prolonged and total sleep deprivation, those specifically attributable to insomnia are limited. People may feel tired, sluggish, inefficient, and more irritable after a poor night's sleep (Zammit, 1988), and these residual effects are more salient in worry-prone individuals (Coyle & Watts, 1991).

VIGNETTE 9.3. Magnifications/Misattributions of Insomnia Consequences

| | |
|---|---|
| *Dysfunctional Cognitions:* | "After a poor night's sleep, I know I won't be able to function the next day." |
| | "When I feel irritable, depressed, or anxious during the day, it is because I haven't slept well the night before." |
| *Underlying Belief:* | "Insomnia is necessarily detrimental to daytime functioning." |
| *Cognitive Errors:* | Misattributions, magnification, overgeneralization. |

*Interventions/Alternative Interpretations:*
(1) Do you *always* experience daytime impairments after a poor night's sleep?
(2) Are these daytime sequelae always experienced with the same intensity?
(3) Is it possible that other factors might also be causing these problems?

However, objective measurements of performance and sleepiness reveal fairly limited residual impairments in unmedicated insomniacs (Stepanski et al., 1988; Stone et al., 1992; Sugerman et al., 1985). The intensity of the subjective complaint about daytime sequelae is often magnified and disproportionate in relation to objective deficits; this is not unlike the amplification of the subjective sleep problem relative to EEG findings. Vignettes 9.3 and 9.4 illustrate these types of misattributions.

Following are examples of how we challenge patients' misattributions and attempt to replace these with more adaptive substitutes:

"Blaming sleep for mood swings, lowered energy, and poor daytime performance is counterproductive. Many other factors, including natural diurnal fluctuations in energy level as well as stress in other areas of your life, may cause those problems. So be careful; don't blame it all on sleep."

VIGNETTE 9.4. Consequences of Insomnia

| | |
|---|---|
| *Dysfunctional Cognition:* | "I am concerned that chronic insomnia may have serious consequences for my physical health." |
| *Underlying Belief:* | "Insomnia is necessarily detrimental to health." |
| *Cognitive Errors:* | Faulty evidence, overgeneralization, catastrophizing. |

*Interventions/Alternative Interpretations:*
(1) There is no evidence that anyone has ever died from lack of sleep alone.
(2) Excessive worrying about insomnia may be more detrimental to health than sleep loss itself.

"Worrying about the daytime consequences of an occasional poor night's sleep only aggravates your problem. Although chronic sleep deprivation impairs functioning, research shows that the performance decrements that can really be traced to insomnia are minimal. When you worry about those presumed consequences, it only makes you more anxious and decreases your tolerance for sleep loss. It also feeds into the vicious cycle of insomnia, emotional distress, and more disturbed sleep."

It is a delicate task to challenge a patient's perceptions of these presumed consequences. Rather than arguing as to whether these daytime sequelae are truly experienced or not, a more fruitful approach is to question the evidence by inquiring whether these problems are experienced every day following a poor night's sleep and whether they are always felt with the same intensity. The patient often agrees that there is indeed some variability; alternative hypotheses that might explain these impairments are then examined. For example, worries stemming from family conflicts, poor time management in the work place, or diminished problem-solving skills in general may interfere with daytime functioning. Yet these difficulties may have been falsely attributed to sleep disturbances. Reattribution training is facilitated by pointing out that nobody functions at peak levels every day, and that within a single day there are variations in performance and mood. Virtually everyone experiences periodic difficulties coping with daily hassles, though not everyone attributes these problems to disturbed sleep. In sum, the patient is encouraged to test alternative hypotheses responsible for daytime impairments and is trained in reattributing perceived sequelae to sources other than insomnia.

## Altering Unrealistic Sleep Expectations

There is a widespread belief that everyone needs 8 hours of sleep every night of the week. For some insomniacs, self-imposed pressure to achieve this "gold standard" creates performance anxiety and exacerbates sleep disturbances. Other insomniacs tend to compare their sleep patterns with those of a friend or bed partner (e.g., "He sleeps like a log"); concerns or worries often arise when the insomniacs realize that they take longer to fall asleep, wake up more often, or simply sleep for shorter durations. Because of individual differences in sleep needs, these variations are not necessarily indicative of insomnia (Lichstein & Fisher, 1985; Morin & Gramling, 1989). Variability can also occur from night to night within a single individual. Examples of unrealistic expectations are presented in Vignettes 9.5 and 9.6.

Cognitive therapy is useful in helping patients distinguish normal from pathological changes in sleep patterns. Simple information about normal developmental changes can alleviate excessive concerns in some individuals

VIGNETTE 9.5. Sleep Requirements Expectations

---

*Dysfunctional Cognition:*      "I must get 8 hours of sleep every night."

*Underlying Belief:*      "It is essential to sleep 8 hours to feel refreshed and function well during the day."

*Cognitive Errors:*      Unrealistic expectation; absolute thinking.

*Interventions/Alternative Interpretations:*
(1) Sleep needs vary widely among individuals, and there is no "gold standard" that everyone should aim for.
(2) Avoid placing undue pressure on yourself to achieve such a standard, as it may increase your anxiety and perpetuate insomnia.
(3) Remember also, that too much sleep may be a waste of time; some very productive people are "short sleepers."

---

and assist them in reappraising the severity and clinical significance of their difficulties. By examining various sleep parameters (e.g., sleep-onset latency, total sleep time) obtained during baseline, the clinician can determine whether these are indicative of a clinical problem or whether they simply fall at the end of the normative range. Sleep diary data can be contrasted with typical cutoff criteria used to define clinical insomnia (e.g., sleep-onset latency or wake after sleep onset > 30 minutes; total sleep time < 6.5 hours). When polysomnographic data are available, they can also be compared to gender- and age-matched normative data (A. Kales & Kales, 1984; Williams et al., 1974). Any variation within these normative ranges should not be considered pathological, inasmuch as there is wide variability across individuals. Here is an example of how we go about altering unrealistic expectations:

VIGNETTE 9.6. Unrealistic Expectations of Self

---

*Dysfunctional Cognition:*      "Because my spouse [significant other] falls asleep in minutes, I should be able to do the same."

*Underlying Belief:*      "Everyone must sleep alike."

*Cognitive Errors:*      Overgeneralization; absolute thinking.

*Interventions/Alternative Interpretations:*
(1) Do all people you know have the same height and weight?
(2) Beyond some normative range, there is wide variability among individuals in terms of how fast they fall asleep, how often they wake up, and the overall quality and duration of sleep.
(3) It is best to avoid social comparisons, as there will always be someone who is wealthier, is taller, and sleeps better than you.

---

"Expectations such as 'I must sleep 8 hours every night' or 'I must fall asleep in minutes' are unrealistic. Although the average sleep duration for adults is between 7½ and 8 hours per night, some people lead very productive lives with as little as 5–6 hours. The speed with which one falls asleep is also variable. Your spouse [partner] may go to sleep as soon as his [her] head hits the pillow, and you may not; still, if you fall asleep in less than 30 minutes, don't worry about it. This is the cutoff criterion to define sleep-onset insomnia. The number and duration of awakenings increase with aging, but these changes are not necessarily indicative of insomnia. The chances are that you wake up more often than you think, inasmuch as you generally don't remember awakenings lasting less than 5 minutes. It is best to avoid comparing your sleep pattern with those of others. There will always be someone who is taller, is wealthier, or sleeps better than you. Simply acknowledge these individual differences and try to remember that you can be just as productive with less time spent asleep."

The main message to communicate here is that a different or changing sleep pattern is not necessarily pathological. The patient is guided to reappraise its clinical meaningfulness. The therapist de-emphasizes social comparisons and encourages the patient to focus on positive attributes for which other people may envy him or her. By pointing out how fortunate some people are to have more time available as a result of their lower sleep requirements, the therapist can even help the patient see how to turn adversity to advantage.

## Enhancing Perceptions of Control and Predictability

There is extensive night-to-night variability in the sleep patterns of insomniacs. This unpredictability tends to reinforce their perception that they have little control over the occurrence of sleep. In turn, decreased self-control is instrumental in producing psychological distress and further sleep difficulties. The typical sequence of events involves anxiety, insomnia, and learned helplessness. For example, individuals with acute insomnia occasionally call in or walk into our clinic in a state of panic, fearing they may never be able to go to sleep again. This excessive fear of losing control is often sparked by a catastrophic apprehension about what may happen if indeed sleep does not come soon. These fears are sufficient to turn what might otherwise have been a transient sleep problem into a chronic one. Over time, performance anxiety and learned helplessness become superimposed on the insomnia problem.

To regain some control and make their sleep somewhat more predictable, insomniacs may engage in a series of prebedtime rituals. In anticipation of a hectic schedule or an important meeting on a given day, they carefully plan the preceding evening and complete all bedtime routines early to ensure that they are in bed by a given time. Although this may seem like a good strategy to facilitate sleep, insomniacs tend to overdo it and develop perform-ance anxiety. Their strong desire to be asleep by a certain time often backfires as the tension builds up throughout the evening and peaks at bedtime. The harder they try, the least successful they are in achieving sleep. Periodic checks of the clock, combined with calculations of how much time is potentially left for sleep, further increase arousal. Vignette 9.7 illustrates this issue of control and performance anxiety.

Two dysfunctional cognitions are present here. One is concerned with the obvious fear of losing control; the other revolves around the presumed effects this might have should it ever happen. First, the therapist attempts to decatastrophize the impact of a sleepless night by inquiring about the most feared consequences. Reappraisal or exaggeration of these consequences may relieve some tension and place insomnia in a more realistic perspective. In addition, clinical use of paradox (i.e., "Try not to sleep; stay up") may foster a patient's sense of personal control; since the patient apparently has little control over sleep, he or she might just as well give it up completely. This paradoxical technique is particularly helpful to alleviate performance anxiety (Ascher & Turner, 1979). Finally, the therapist can say something like the following:

"Catastrophizing after a sleepless night only makes matters worse. Sleep loss is more likely to be distressing if you perceive it as stressful than if you see it as a challenge. So don't panic after a sleepless night; stay calm and accept the fact you didn't sleep well the night before. The only certain consequence of sleeplessness is that it will eventual-ly lead to sleepiness."

Learned helplessness is the next target for intervention, and causal attributions are particularly important here. The lack of explanation for a

**VIGNETTE 9.7.** Diminished Control over Sleep and Performance Anxiety

| | |
|---|---|
| *Dysfunctional Cognitions*: | "I am afraid of losing control over my sleep abilities." "I have lost control of my sleep." |
| *Underlying Belief*: | "It is essential to be in full control of all aspects of one's life." |
| *Cognitive Errors*: | Catastrophizing; irrational belief. |

*Interventions/Alternative Interpretations*:
(1) What is the worst thing that could happen if you never got to sleep tonight? It is not catastrophic to go without sleep.
(2) The harder you try to control sleep, the less control you will achieve; it is much easier to force wakefulness than to fall asleep at will.
(3) Sleep will come more easily if you do not try so hard to control it.

sleepless night is often the most distressing aspect of insomnia; it reinforces the personal conviction that sleep is unpredictable. On the other hand, when insomnia is attributed strictly to external factors, a natural response is to rely on sleep aids to make sleep more predictable. This scenario is typical of chronic insomniacs who present in therapy with undue pessimism and a perception of having little control over their natural sleep-inducing abilities, both of which have led to and been reinforced by long-term use of hypnotic medications. Vignette 9.8 illustrates these issues.

The intervention targets both causal attributions and perceived lack of control. For example, if insomnia is primarily attributed to a chemical imbalance, medication is likely to be seen as the only effective treatment. When medication is used on a sporadic basis (e.g., "only when I really need to be up to par the next day"), tolerance to the drug is minimized and its efficacy is prolonged. In turn, prolonged efficacy may only confirm the patient's perception of having little control over his or her natural sleep-inducing abilities. The intervention must focus on breaking this circular reasoning. To foster self-efficacy, the patient must be trained to identify possible causes responsible for his or her insomnia. A careful review of activities, concerns, and worries of the previous day/evening almost always uncovers some reasons why sleep was disturbed on that night. Viewing a poor night's sleep as the result of specific daytime stressors, or simply as the result of worrying too much about sleeplessness, is more adaptive than interpreting it as further evidence of lack of control.

---

**VIGNETTE 9.8.** Unpredictability of Sleep and Learned Helplessness

---

| | |
|---|---|
| *Dysfunctional Cognitions:* | "I usually can't predict whether I'll have a good or poor night's sleep." |
| | "I must rely on a sleeping aid to make my sleep more predictable." |
| *Underlying Belief:* | "No matter what I do, it has no effect on sleep. Insomnia is mostly a result of external factors that I have little control over. I am a victim." |
| *Cognitive Errors:* | Overgeneralization, faulty evidence, circular reasoning. |

*Interventions/Alternative Interpretations:*

(1) When you use a sleeping pill and experience some temporary relief, it only reinforces your conviction that you have little control over sleep.

(2) Nighttime sleep is not independent of daytime activities, thoughts, and feelings; therefore, you must carefully examine these relationships in order to make your sleep more predictable and develop more self-control.

(3) Remember also that the most predictable consequence of sleeplessness is that it will eventually lead to sleepiness.

---

VIGNETTE 9.9. Excessive Emphasis on Sleep and Control

---

*Dysfunctional Cognitions*:            "I feel insomnia is destroying my entire life."
                                       "I have little control in managing the negative con-
                                       sequences of disturbed sleep."

*Underlying Belief*:                   "I am helpless/hopeless; unless sleep improves, my life
                                       will remain miserable."

*Cognitive Errors*:                    Magnification; overgeneralization; catastrophizing.

*Interventions/Alternative Interpretations*:
(1) Since sleep is supposed to occupy only a third of your life, aren't you giving it more
    importance than it deserves?
(2) Is it possible the next time you have a bad night's sleep to ignore it and go about your daily
    routines just pretending you slept well?

---

For some chronic insomniacs, sleep is the essence of their existence. Their social, recreational, occupational, and family activities are all contingent upon the quality and duration of their sleep. In turn, this excessive emphasis on sleep strengthens the belief that insomnia is destroying their entire lives. Vignette 9.9 exemplifies this issue.

Such patients are taught to develop some tolerance to sleep loss and to its perceived sequelae. Although it is important to recognize that insomnia does indeed diminish the quality of life, it should not be allowed to control it entirely. Taking time off from work or canceling social/family commitments because of poor sleep may serve as a secondary gain and provide negative reinforcement for the insomnia process. It is essential to motivate patients to go on with their usual daily routines and planned schedules, regardless of how they slept. Recommending a pleasant activity contingent upon a poor night's sleep may enhance the perception that adequate functioning is still possible with insomnia. The main message to convey here is that patients can still lead satisfactory lives despite sleep difficulties; they are not helpless.

Control and predictability, or the lack thereof, are two core features of insomnia. These issues become particularly relevant during the maintenance phase of therapy. It may take a series of good nights' sleep before a patient regains a sense of control and feels more self-efficacious. Even after the sleep pattern has been stabilized, occasional setbacks are common. To prevent a relapse, the patient must come to see these occasional bad nights as either natural or resulting from identifiable causes (e.g., stress at work, conflicts with spouse), rather than as evidence of loss of control. Developing greater tolerance to these few bad nights is very important. The patient must learn to remain calm and go on with the usual routines, rather than catastrophizing and assuming that chronic insomnia has returned.

**VIGNETTE 9.10.** Misconceptions about Good Sleep Practices

| | |
|---|---|
| *Dysfunctional Cognition:* | "When I don't get an adequate amount of sleep, I need to catch up by sleeping late the next morning or by napping the next day." |
| *Underlying Belief:* | "It is essential to make up for all sleep loss." |
| *Cognitive Errors:* | Faulty evidence; absolute thinking. |

*Interventions/Alternative Interpretations:*

(1) Sleeping too late in the morning or taking daytime naps is likely to delay sleep onset the next night.

(2) Sleep deprivation experiments have shown that people only need to make up for about one-third of previous sleep loss.

## Dispelling Myths about Good Sleep Practices

Just as people hold faulty beliefs about the causes and consequences of their insomnia, they may also entertain preconceived ideas about sleep-promoting practices. Insomniacs often believe that the best way to get to sleep is to stay in bed and try harder, or that the best coping strategy to minimize the consequences of sleep loss is to take daytime naps. These practices perpetuate sleep difficulties, regardless of how strong the underlying belief is. Vignettes 9.10, 9.11, and 9.12 illustrate faulty beliefs specifically related to sleep-promoting practices.

Most of these faulty beliefs have already been addressed directly through the introduction of stimulus control and sleep restriction. It may be important to review these concepts again with the patient to strengthen the position that

**VIGNETTE 9.11.** Other Misconceptions about Good Sleep Practices

| | |
|---|---|
| *Dysfunctional Cognition:* | "When I have trouble sleeping, I should just stay in bed and try harder." |
| *Underlying Belief:* | "If I get out of bed, I will wake up even more and surely won't be able to go back to sleep." |
| *Cognitive Errors:* | Faulty assumption/evidence. |

*Interventions/Alternative Interpretations:*

(1) The harder you try to induce sleep at will, the less likely you are to succeed. Have you ever noticed that you fall asleep unintentionally when you are not even trying (e.g., reading, watching TV)?

(2) When you stay in bed awake for too long, it only strengthens the association between your sleep surroundings and tension/frustration.

**VIGNETTE 9.12.** Further Misconceptions about Good Sleep Practices

| | |
|---|---|
| *Dysfunctional Cognition:* | "If I just spend more time in bed, I will eventually get all the sleep/rest I need." |
| *Underlying Belief:* | "Lying down in bed, even if I am awake, provides some very needed rest." |
| *Cognitive Errors:* | Faulty evidence/assumption. |

*Interventions/Alternative Interpretations:*
(1) Have you ever paid close attention to the way you feel after spending 12 hours in bed? Do you really feel good and refreshed upon arising?
(2) It is best to spend less time in bed and sleep more efficiently.

these behavioral patterns are maladaptive and unhealthy. A didactic approach may be sufficient for some people to modify these faulty beliefs, whereas others may require a more systematic cognitive restructuring intervention.

## Clinical Issues and Problems

The relative importance of each of the five types of dysfunctional cognitions outlined above will vary among patients, according to their own personal and learning histories. It is therefore essential to identify the most clinically relevant areas for each patient and to target those for intervention. Several problematic issues may arise in the process of implementing cognitive restructuring techniques.

First, a word of caution is in order for clinicians unfamiliar with insomnia. It is particularly important to avoid the argument that insomnia has no impact on daytime functioning and that all sequelae reported by patients are figments of their imagination. Although chronic insomnia produces limited daytime residual deficits, it can still be very debilitating for some individuals. The main difference between poor and good sleepers seems to be the relative emphasis placed by these two groups on sleeplessness and its consequences. Insomniacs tend to catastrophize over temporary sleep loss and to amplify its negative impact on daytime functioning. Thus, the clinician must on the one hand show strong empathy and support, but on the other hand must skillfully use cognitive restructuring techniques (reattribution, decatastrophizing, attention shifting, etc.). Also, because most health care professionals have themselves experienced situational insomnia at some time in their lives, it is important for a therapist to be aware of his or her own preconceived notions regarding the causes and consequences of chronic insomnia (Pressman, 1991).

Second, confronting the patient's ideas and beliefs about sleeplessness is a delicate task, since these are usually well ingrained at the time of treatment. For this reason, implementation of cognitive restructuring techniques requires sophisticated clinical skills. For example, a patient recently brought in a newspaper story reporting on a few cases of fatal familial insomnia in Italy, in order to convince his therapist that he could indeed die of insomnia. These extremely rare cases proved to be related to an underlying neurological disorder. Nevertheless, such an example of selective abstraction will require a very skillful therapist to bring solid and credible arguments to counteract the dysfunctional belief. Furthermore, it is essential to confront the ideas and beliefs, not the patient. Some individuals may still be offended; as a result they may well become resistant and defensive, and may withdraw from the therapeutic exchange. Ongoing monitoring of these reactions is essential, as well as periodic assessment of each patient's acceptance and understanding of cognitive therapy premises.

Finally, cognitive therapy is essentially a technique of verbal persuasion. Some patients will respond to simple education, whereas others will require a great deal more therapeutic effort. Implementation of this therapy component is generally more time-consuming, and requires more training and experience on the part of the clinician, than implementation of the behavioral and sleep hygiene components.

## Conclusion

Insomnia sufferers come to therapy with their own cognitive sets made up of beliefs, expectations, and attributions. Whereas some of these cognitions are valid and adaptive, others will prove faulty and maladaptive, and will be found to feed into the insomnia problem. These dysfunctional sleep cognitions represent important targets for treatment. There is already an extensive literature on the role of cognitive variables in mediating conceptually similar disorders (e.g., anxiety and affective disorders) and on the efficacy of cognitive therapy in alleviating these dysfunctions. Although data specific to insomniac populations are still limited, a few preliminary treatment studies specifically targeting dysfunctional beliefs and attitudes (Edinger et al., 1992; Morin, Stone, et al., 1992; Morin, Kowatch, et al., 1993; Sanavio, 1988; Sanavio et al., 1990) have provided encouraging results supporting the use of cognitive interventions for the successful management of insomnia.

# 10

Sleep Hygiene Education

Sleep is affected by a host of lifestyle and environmental factors, including diet, exercise, alcohol, and substance use, as well as noise, light, and temperature. These various factors, which may be beneficial or detrimental to sleep, are usually referred to as "sleep hygiene" (Hauri, 1982). Some clinicians also include in this rubric other maladaptive habits, such as daytime napping, variable sleep scheduling, excessive time spent in bed, sleep-incompatible activities, and inadequate prebedtime routines. These latter behaviors, however, have led to well-specified procedures (e.g., stimulus control, sleep restriction) and are covered in other chapters. In the interest of treatment specificity, sleep hygiene in the present context is limited to two elements: (1) health practices (i.e., diet, exercise, and substance use) and (2) environmental influences (i.e., light, noise, temperature, and mattress). This chapter reviews these factors and outlines a series of clinical guidelines to safeguard against their interference with sleep.

## Sleep Hygiene and Insomnia

Clinicians and laypeople alike often speculate about the effects of various health habits on sleep. For example, it is generally assumed that caffeine disrupts sleep and that physical exercise improves its quality. Clinical recommendations for insomnia often require that people discontinue caffeine, quit smoking, or enroll in an aerobics class. Research conducted with good sleepers indicate that caffeine (Karacan et al., 1976) and nicotine (Soldatos, Kales, Scharf, Bixler, & Kales, 1980) do indeed disrupt sleep, whereas exercise may deepen it (Horne, 1981; Torsvall, 1981). The lifestyle of insomniacs is generally more sedentary than that of good sleepers (Marchini et al., 1983). A comparison of these two groups on sleep hygiene knowledge and practices also reveals that insomniacs are better informed but engage in more unhealthy habits than good sleepers (Lacks & Rotert, 1986).

Little information is yet available on the clinical effectiveness of interventions directly manipulating these health practices among poor sleepers. For instance, no studies have evaluated the impact of a structured aerobic exercise on the sleep patterns of chronic insomniacs. Similarly, there are few data on the effect of discontinuing caffeine intake in poor sleepers. Although most interventions incorporate education to safeguard against interference from these factors (Engle-Friedman et al., 1992; Schoicket et al., 1988), sleep hygiene as the sole treatment for insomnia has yielded limited benefits (Lacks & Morin, 1992; Morin & Kwentus, 1988). For example, in a study specifically addressing this issue, sleep hygiene produced a modest 27% reduction in time spent awake after sleep onset, and patient satisfaction was significantly lower with this intervention than with other treatment modalities (e.g., stimulus control and meditation) (Schoicket et al., 1988). These limited therapeutic gains may be explained by the fact that inadequate sleep hygiene is rarely the primary cause of insomnia, and that it reaches sufficient severity to produce insomnia in only a few patients (Reynolds et al., 1991). Nevertheless, because these factors may complicate or exacerbate an existing problem and hinder treatment progress, it is important to examine their relative contribution to insomnia and to integrate sleep hygiene education into the overall intervention.

## Treatment Goals and Rationale

The objectives of sleep hygiene education are twofold: (1) to heighten the patient's awareness and knowledge of the impact of health-related habits and environmental factors on sleep; and (2) to promote better sleep hygiene practices. After the initial evaluation, the clinician should already have some notions of the patient's sleep hygiene and its relative contributory role to insomnia (see sections 5 and 6 of the Insomnia Interview Schedule [Appendix A]). A more detailed evaluation of these factors can be obtained with the Sleep Hygiene Awareness and Practice Scale, a 50-item questionnaire tapping both knowledge and practices of various activities/substances either beneficial or disruptive to sleep (Lacks & Rotert, 1986).

In the following sections, I review those factors with the greatest potential for inhibiting or facilitating sleep. The empirical evidence documenting their impact on sleep is summarized, and clinical guidelines to improve sleep hygiene practices are reviewed. This treatment component is primarily educational in nature and involves mostly didactic teaching. The clinician's role is to (1) review each of these principles; (2) gauge the patient's knowledge about it; (3) present basic facts to correct misconceptions or reinforce correct knowledge; and (4) make appropriate behavior change recommendations.

Several sleep hygiene rules are outlined in Table 10.1, which can be given as a handout to patients (though it is sometimes best to select only those procedures directly relevant to a given patient).

## Caffeine

Caffeine is the most widely used drug in our society. It is a central nervous system stimulant and is often used to promote alertness. Depending on its preparation, one cup of coffee contains between 100 and 200 mg of caffeine, while tea and soft drinks (e.g., Pepsi, Coke) contain between 50 and 75 mg. Caffeine reaches its peak plasma levels within 1 hour (15–45 minutes) of intake. Its half-life elimination, which shows considerable variation between individuals, ranges from 3 to 7 hours (Curatolo & Robertson, 1983). Caffeine is also contained in cocoa, chocolate, and various over-the-counter medications (e.g., anorectic, allergy, and cold remedies). Bedtime use of these products can have the same detrimental effects as coffee on nocturnal sleep.

Caffeine is a potent sleep inhibitor. Laboratory studies have shown that when it is consumed within 30 to 60 minutes of bedtime, caffeine increases sleep latency and night wakings, decreases total sleep time and slow-wave sleep, and impairs subjective sleep quality (Karacan et al., 1976). There is a dose-related effect, with one cup of coffee having minimal impact and two to four cups producing significant sleep disruptions in otherwise good sleepers. Although few people drink two to four cups of coffee just before bedtime, it is not unusual to see patients consuming caffeine products (e.g., soft drinks, iced tea, chocolate) almost continually throughout the evening. Moderate daytime consumption is unlikely to affect nighttime sleep, but its heavy use

---

**TABLE 10.1.** Sleep Hygiene Guidelines

---

1. Caffeine is a stimulant and should be discontinued 4–6 hours before bedtime.

2. Nicotine is also a stimulant and should be avoided near bedtime and upon night wakings.

3. Alcohol is a depressant; although it may facilitate sleep onset, it causes awakenings later in the night.

4. A light snack may be sleep-inducing, but a heavy meal too close to bedtime interferes with sleep.

5. Do not exercise vigorously within 3–4 hours of bedtime; regular exercise in the late afternoon may deepen sleep.

6. Minimize noise, light, and excessive temperature during the sleep period with ear plugs, window blinds, or an electric blanket/air conditioner.

---

throughout the day may be followed by evening withdrawal symptoms (e.g., headaches), which can inhibit sleep onset (Hughes et al., 1991).

Sensitivity and tolerance to caffeine may vary across individuals and produce different effects on sleep. J. D. Kales et al. (1984) found no difference in caffeine intake between poor and good sleepers; however, insomniacs may be more sensitive to its stimulating effects, owing to a greater predisposition to hyperarousal. A higher tolerance may also explain why some habitual caffeine consumers do not complain of insomnia, whereas moderate consumers or nonconsumers report sleep disturbances after a single cup of coffee (Levy & Zylber-Katz, 1983). In general, caffeine disturbs objective sleep parameters even in those who subjectively claim that it has no impact on theirs.

Despite the extensive empirical evidence confirming caffeine's powerful sleep-altering effect, only one study has evaluated the impact of discontinuing caffeine intake on sleep patterns (Edelstein, Keaton-Brasted, & Burg, 1984). This naturalistic study showed that elimination of caffeine in 10 psychiatric inpatients with sleep-maintenance insomnia decreased the frequency of night wakings and reduced the number of requests for sleep medication. In summary, the empirical evidence supports the popular notion that caffeine interferes with sleep and that its elimination may improve sleep. Because of its relatively long half-life, caffeine should be discontinued at least 4–6 hours prior to bedtime.

## Nicotine

Nicotine is also a central nervous system stimulant and produces much the same effects as caffeine on sleep. Although many individuals claim that smoking helps them to relax, the overall effect of nicotine is one of stimulation rather than relaxation. At low blood concentrations nicotine may produce a mild and very brief sedation, but with higher blood levels this state is rapidly replaced by physiological arousal (i.e., increased heart rate, blood pressure, and catecholamine concentration). The net result is one of autonomic activation, which is associated with problems in initiating and sustaining sleep. The stimulating effects of caffeine and nicotine are additive and are particularly detrimental to sleep.

Surveys and laboratory studies have confirmed the association between smoking and sleep difficulties. Those smoking more than one pack per day have significantly more difficulty falling asleep than either nonsmokers or those smoking less than a pack per day (J. D. Kales et al., 1984). Smokers take longer to fall asleep and have a lower sleep efficiency than nonsmokers (Soldatos et al., 1980). Excessive smoking near bedtime may lead to conditioned arousals in the night. In heavy smokers, for example, the first thought upon waking in the middle of the night is often to smoke a cigarette.

With repeated occurrences, sleep interruptions may become conditioned to nicotine withdrawal.

Smoking cessation improved the sleep patterns of eight chronic cigarette smokers (Soldatos et al., 1980). Sleep induction was shortened on the first three nights, and sleep maintenance was strengthened beginning on the fourth and fifth nights subsequent to smoking cessation. These changes are particularly meaningful because they occurred in spite of the daytime withdrawal symptoms associated with smoking cessation. Unfortunately, no other study has investigated the impact of smoking cessation on the duration, efficiency, or quality of sleep.

To summarize, nicotine has a stimulating effect that is associated with problems in initiating and sustaining sleep. Smoking cessation is followed by reduced sleep-onset latency and time awake after sleep onset. The best advice is obviously to quit the smoking habit altogether. For patients who cannot or will not kick the habit, it is particularly important to reduce the rate of smoking prior to bedtime. To prevent further strengthening of conditioned awakenings to nicotine withdrawal, patients should be firmly instructed to avoid smoking when waking up in the middle of the night.

## Alcohol

Unlike caffeine and nicotine, alcohol is a central nervous system depressant; nonetheless, it is the substance most likely to cause sleep disruption. Alcohol is metabolized at approximately the rate of one drink per hour, and the withdrawal effects may persist for 2–4 hours even after the blood level has returned to zero. Even a moderate and socially acceptable amount of alcohol between dinner and bedtime is likely to disrupt nocturnal sleep.

Alcohol consumed near bedtime hastens sleep onset and deepens sleep in the first part of the night; however, the overall effect is one of sleep fragmentation. As the alcohol is metabolized, withdrawal symptoms occur, and sleep becomes interrupted and shortened. Acute presleep alcohol intake suppresses REM sleep early in the night and is followed by a REM rebound in the latter part of the night. Early-morning awakenings are often triggered by nightmares, which themselves are associated with excessive REM activity occurring in the second half of the night (Zarcone, 1989).

The effects of chronic alcohol abuse on sleep are even more pronounced (Mendelson, 1987). Following a binge episode, sleep may initially be deeper, but difficulties in sustaining it are common. With acute withdrawal, sleep is fragmented, shallow, and shortened; there is also a marked reduction of stages 3–4, as well as a slight decrease in REM sleep (Johnson, Burdick, & Smith, 1970). During prolonged abstinence, the percentage of stages 3–4 remains diminished, stage 1 is increased, and sleep interruptions are more frequent

(Snyder & Karacan, 1985). Behavioral and dietary factors often interact with alcohol abuse in altering the circadian rhythm and the sleep–wake cycle.

For social drinkers or those using an occasional nightcap as a sleeping aid, the best advice is to avoid alcoholic beverages for 4–6 hours prior to bedtime. Although a drink may help anxious insomniacs to relax and fall asleep more quickly, alcohol is particularly detrimental to sleep continuity. For alcoholics, treatment should first be directed at the underlying substance abuse problem. However, even among recovered substance abusers, severe insomnia may persist for extensive periods of time and may precipitate relapse. Cognitive-behavioral therapy may be useful during this stage to minimize the risks of relapse that are specifically attributable to pervasive sleep disturbances.

## Diet

Little research has systematically evaluated the effects of dietary habits on sleep. Aside from clinical observations that a meal high in carbohydrates promotes sleepiness and that one high in protein enhances alertness, claims that various diets promote human sleep are for the most part unsubstantiated. Food intake by itself may be sleep–inducing, but both the timing and the amount of caloric intake are important mediating factors (Adam, 1980). For example, a light snack at bedtime seems to promote sleep, though this prebedtime routine may well serve as a discriminative stimulus that becomes conditioned to drowsiness. On the other hand, a heavy meal at bedtime is contraindicated, as it activates the digestive system and interferes with sleep. Interestingly, the sleepiness commonly experienced in midafternoon is more strongly associated with a circadian factor (i.e., a slight drop in body temperature) than with food intake alone.

Clinical evidence suggests that milk and other dairy products are sleep-promoting. L-Tryptophan, a natural amino acid found in milk and in many other foods, is a precursor of the neurotransmitter serotonin, whose concentration is increased during sleep. Although it should theoretically promote sleep, empirical findings with human subjects have been inconsistent. Some studies have reported improved sleep (Hartmann, 1977), whereas others have shown no effects with 2, 4, or even 6 grams of L-tryptophan (Nicholson & Stone, 1979a). A major problem with these studies, however, is that they have generally been conducted with volunteers who are already good sleepers at baseline, leaving little room for further improvement.

L-Tryptophan was available until recently in most health food stores. A recent investigation by the Food and Drug Administration (FDA) and the Centers for Disease Control (CDC) has linked this amino acid with eosinophilia, a blood disease associated with an increase of white blood cells.

Several patients who had been using this food supplement contracted this disease, which proved fatal in some cases. More recent investigations suggest that this disease was not directly linked to L-tryptophan, but instead resulted from other contaminating substances inadvertently introduced in the process of manufacturing a few batches of this food supplement. Nevertheless, the FDA has since recommended that L-tryptophan be withdrawn from the market. This is somewhat unfortunate, because this natural hypnotic serves as an excellent temporary substitute while drug-dependent insomniacs are being tapered off their prescribed sleeping pills. The specific effects of dairy products on sleep are uncertain, as their tryptophan content is much lower than that available in concentrated pills.

Changes in body weight are often associated with alterations of sleep patterns. For instance, weight loss is accompanied by short and fragmented sleep, whereas weight gain is associated with long and continuous sleep. Thyroid functions may mediate these changes. Hyperthyroidism results in weight loss and short but deep sleep; hypothyroidism is linked with weight gain and long but lighter sleep (A. Kales & Kales, 1984). Patients enrolled in weight reduction programs frequently report problems in falling asleep or staying asleep (Crisp, Stonehill, Fenton, & Fenwick, 1973). Likewise, anorectic patients experience sleep-maintenance difficulties, and their sleep generally improves following weight gain (Lacey, Crisp, Kalucy, Hartmann, & Chen, 1975). It is unclear whether changes in sleep patterns are more strongly related to nutritional deficiencies than to mood disturbances. In depressed patients, weight loss is associated with insomnia, whereas weight gain is linked with hypersomnia.

On the basis of current evidence, a light snack with a nonalcoholic and noncaffeinated beverage before bedtime may be sleep-promoting in some individuals. Although it is best to avoid going to bed hungry, a heavy meal before bedtime is contraindicated. Snacks in the middle of the night should be discouraged, as night wakings may become conditioned to hunger. Excessive fluid intake in the evening should also be avoided, as it may lead to nocturia and problems in returning to sleep. This is particularly important for older adults, who are more prone to bladder problems and who may already use diuretics.

## Exercise

The benefits of aerobic exercise on health and physical fitness have been well studied and are relatively well understood. The impact of exercise on sleep is more equivocal (Horne, 1981; Torsvall, 1981). Sleep is assumed to serve several functions, including that of physical energy restoration. Recovery from fatigue has been attributed specifically to slow-wave sleep (stages 3 and

4). According to this restorative theory, physical activity should increase total sleep time and slow-wave sleep. It is also commonly assumed that running, swimming, skiing, or any activities resulting in energy expenditure promote deep sleep, though empirical evidence on this issue is controversial.

Three factors seem to mediate the relationship between physical exercise and sleep: the amount of energy expenditure, the timing of physical activity in relation to the sleep period, and a subject's initial physical fitness. Several studies have reported a decrease in sleep-onset latency and an increase in slow-wave and total sleep following sustained exercise in physically fit individuals (Browman, 1980; Bunnell, Bevier, & Horvath, 1983; Griffin & Trinder, 1978; Shapiro, Bortz, Mitchell, Bartel, & Jooste, 1981). Other investigations have failed to confirm these findings with untrained subjects, for whom sleep following sustained exercise was more fragmented and restless (see Horne, 1981). Thus, physical fitness is an important factor in determining whether exercise has any benefits on sleep. The timing of exercise in relation to the sleep period is equally important. Exercising just before bedtime produces a "stress effect" and elevates autonomic activity, which in turn causes restlessness, increased wakefulness and stage 1 sleep, and decreased slow-wave sleep (Torsvall, 1981). Conversely, physical exercise in the morning may have minimal impact on nighttime sleep because of the too-distant temporal relationship. Perhaps the best time to exercise is in late afternoon or early evening, because the rebound cooling occurring a few hours later is conducive to sleep (Horne & Staff, 1983). Finally, the amount of energy expenditure is also an important variable mediating the relationship between exercise and sleep. Running a marathon affects sleep differently than does jogging for 30 minutes. Strenuous exercise is likely to disrupt sleep on the following night even in the most physically fit individual.

What are the implications of these findings for the treatment of sleep complaints? Should exercise be recommended as a cure for insomnia? As for most sleep hygiene factors, no study has evaluated the effects of a regular exercise program on the sleep of insomniacs. This is an important research question, particularly for older insomniacs. Age is a major factor associated with decreased slow-wave sleep; theoretically, exercise should promote retention of this deep sleep. Although some data suggest that exercise frequency alone does not discriminate between older adults with and without insomnia complaints (Morin & Gramling, 1989), a more adequate measure (e.g., the amount of daily energy expenditure) might yield different results.

On the basis of the current empirical evidence on exercise and sleep, two clinical recommendations can safely be made. First, insomnia sufferers should avoid vigorous exercise too close to bedtime, as this accentuates autonomic arousal and causes restless sleep. Second, they should be encouraged to enroll in a regular exercise program in late afternoon or early evening, not only as a sleep-promoting activity but also as a general stress reduction method.

## Noise, Light, Temperature, and Mattress

Environmental factors such as noise, room temperature, light, and mattress comfort can interfere with sleep. A comfortable bed in a quiet and darkened room free from extreme temperatures does not necessarily guarantee sound sleep; however, any disruption in these environmental conditions is likely to interfere with normal sleep. Sensitivity to these factors is variable among individuals. While some people can adjust to almost any sleep environment, others often develop transient insomnia in strange surroundings.

Noise from a crying baby, a snoring bedmate, or street traffic can delay sleep onset or cause awakenings. The awakening threshold is lowest in stage 1 sleep, highest in stages 3–4 sleep, and variable in REM sleep. The meaningfulness of the auditory stimuli influences this threshold; for instance, a new parent will be awakened more easily by a crying baby than by street noise. The awakening threshold decreases with aging, and it may account for the increased prevalence of sleep-maintenance insomnia in late life. A noise level sufficient to wake up a 70-year-old causes only a temporary shift to light sleep in a 25-year-old (Parkes, 1985). Although people may habituate to noise from street traffic, their sleep remains shallower and lighter. The increased subjective sensitivity to noise in insomniacs is consistent with their higher autonomic arousal and chronic state of hypervigilance.

Although there is no ideal room temperature for everyone, exposure to extreme temperatures interferes with normal sleep. A hot room (above 24°C/ 75°F) increases night wakings, reduces REM and delta sleep, causes more body movements and shifts in sleep stages, and impairs the overall quality of sleep (Libert et al., 1991). Although sleep difficulties are less frequently associated with cold rooms, a decrease in room temperature below 12°C (54°F) leads to more unpleasant and more emotional dreams (Hauri, 1982).

Body temperature also influences sleep. Poor sleepers often report being hotter than good sleepers, which is consistent with their elevated body temperature observed throughout the 24-hour cycle. The rebound cooling following active (exercise) or passive (hot bath) body heating is conducive to sleep, and this cooling occurs earlier with passive than with active heating (Bunnell, Agnew, Horvath, Jopson, & Wills, 1988; Horne & Staff, 1983). This phenomena explains in part why insomniacs should not engage in vigorous exercise within 3–4 hours of bedtime, whereas they might take a hot bath up to 2 hours before bedtime.

Excessive lighting and a poor mattress are two additional environmental factors that may disturb sleep. Although firmness of mattress is often a matter of personal preference, a mattress that is too hard may cause sleep difficulties in those with arthritis, whereas one that is too soft may be problematic for patients with low back pain. Excessive lighting conditions can cause trouble sleeping in almost anyone, and this factor alone may exacerbate the already high prevalence of insomnia in night workers trying to sleep by day.

Several simple environmental changes can reduce the impact of the physical surroundings on sleep behaviors (Morin & Rapp, 1987). First, it is particularly important to ensure a well-darkened room, with window shades preventing street lights or daylight from coming through the windows. Strategic placement of curtains or a change from global to spot lightning can reduce undesired illumination in some environments. On the other hand, individuals whose insomnia is attributable to jet lag, night work, or other circadian disruptions may benefit from light therapy (Allen, 1991; Czeisler et al., 1990). The use of a background noise from a fan or "white noise" from a radio can mask more disruptive sounds. Ear plugs will significantly reduce the noise level, as will a better-insulated room. Temperature is more easily adjusted with the use of blankets for a cold environment or air conditioning for a warm room. An excessively soft mattress can be made firmer by placing boards beneath it, though it may be necessary to replace it altogether.

Needless to say, individuals living in their own homes or apartments have more control over their sleep environments than do hospitalized or institutionalized persons. Bedmates may need to adjust to each other's preferences, but for the most part these environmental changes are fairly easy to implement. Conversely, personal control over environmental factors is substantially reduced in inpatient settings (residential, institutional, and hospital), and sleep disturbances attributable to noise, lighting, room temperature, and uncomfortable mattresses are extremely prevalent in these settings (Berlin, 1984).

## Clinical Issues and Problems

Sleep is a topic of popular interest and receives extensive media coverage. Insomniacs are particularly avid readers of articles on the subject and are generally well informed about the impact of various lifestyles and environmental factors on sleep. Even though most sleep hygiene principles are matters of common sense, the clinician should not assume that patients adhere to them consistently. As noted earlier, insomniacs may be better informed but may generally engage in more unhealthy practices than good sleepers (Lacks & Rotert, 1986). In addition, many insomniacs feel that they are "immune" to these factors and continue to engage in detrimental practices until specifically instructed otherwise.

The clinician should systematically inquire about lifestyle and environmental factors, examine their relative contribution to insomnia, and make appropriate recommendations. Even obvious-seeming factors should not be overlooked. For example, caffeine intake should be examined closely and self-monitored when necessary. Some patients claim that they never drink coffee after dinner, yet in the evening they may consume several caffeinated soft drinks and eat chocolate. A snoring bedmate may also be very disruptive to someone sensitive to noise, though some people are reluctant to complain about this. Finally, some individuals are so accustomed to sleeping in poor environmental conditions that they are unaware of their detrimental impact; others are simply reluctant to admit such poor conditions to the therapist. When such factors are salient enough to be the primary causes of insomnia, it is best to alter the sequence of the various treatment components. Sleep hygiene education should then be introduced prior to implementing the behavioral and cognitive components.

As for all therapy components, the clinician should give patients a handout of the treatment procedure (see Table 10.1). This will enhance recall, understanding, and integration of the clinical procedures. It is important to remember however, that some patients will focus on those procedures that are irrelevant for them, and minimize those that are most clinically relevant. As such, it may be best to give a written description only of those procedures most relevant for a given patient.

## Conclusion

Education and promotion of better sleep hygiene practices play an important role in the management of insomnia. Various lifestyle and environmental conditions may have a direct detrimental effect on nocturnal sleep or may interact with other factors to complicate insomnia. Although inadequate sleep hygiene in itself is rarely the primary cause of insomnia, it may hinder progress and interfere with clinical efforts to modify other maladaptive behavior patterns and dysfunctional cognitions. From a clinical perspective, sleep hygiene education is a necessary component to safeguard against interference from these factors; as the sole intervention, however, it may produce limited benefits and is best integrated into a multifaceted intervention program.

# 11

## Sleep Medications

This chapter addresses the pharmacological management of insomnia and withdrawal from sleep medications. The first section presents an overview of drugs commonly prescribed for insomnia. Their effects on sleep and daytime functioning are summarized, and relative indications and contraindications are outlined. The second section describes a withdrawal program for drug-dependent insomniacs. Pharmacotherapy is the most frequently used method for treating insomnia; however, it may also lead to iatrogenic insomnia. Most importantly, chronic use of sleep medications undermines the development of appropriate self-management skills to cope with insomnia.

### Pharmacotherapy

Several classes of medications are used in the management of insomnia: benzodiazepines, barbiturates, nonbenzodiazepine hypnotics, antidepressants, and over-the-counter sleep aids. Barbiturates such as secobarbital (Seconal), amobarbital (Amytal), and pentobarbital (Nembutal) are potent hypnotics, but their use has been almost completely abandoned because of their higher level of toxicity, interaction with other drugs, and higher risks for tolerance and dependence. Likewise, other compounds (e.g., meprobamate, chloral hydrate, and glutethimide) are no longer indicated in the management of insomnia because of higher risks of drug interactions.

### Benzodiazepines

The benzodiazepines are recognized as the treatment of choice when a sleep medication is deemed clinically indicated (National Institutes of Health [NIH], 1984). Although most benzodiazepines have sedative and hypnotic properties, only five of them are marketed as hypnotics in the United States (see Table 11.1). Their main differences are based on their pharmacokinetic

TABLE 11.1. Pharmacokinetics and Dosage of Benzodiazepine Hypnotics

| Generic name | Trade name | Absorption | Half-life (hours) | Dosage (milligrams) |
|---|---|---|---|---|
| Estazolam | ProSom | Rapid | 8–24 | 1.0–2.0 |
| Flurazepam | Dalmane | Rapid | 48–120 | 15.0–30.0 |
| Quazepam | Doral | Rapid | 48–120 | 15.0–30.0 |
| Temazepam | Restoril | Intermediate | 8–20 | 7.5–30.0 |
| Triazolam | Halcion | Rapid | 2–6 | 0.125–0.25 |

properties: absorption, distribution, and elimination. The rate of absorption and rate of distribution determine the speed of onset of the drug effect; elimination half-life and rate of distribution determine the length of time during which drug effects persist. Combined with the dosage, these properties mediate the effects of the drugs on sleep and on daytime functioning (Greenblatt, 1991).

All benzodiazepine hypnotics are effective in the short-term management of insomnia. Compared to placebo, they reduce sleep-onset latency, decrease the number and duration of nocturnal awakenings, and increase total sleep time and sleep efficiency (A. Kales, Bixler, Kales, & Scharf, 1977; Morin & Kwentus, 1988; Mendelson, 1987). Selection of a particular agent is partly dependent on the nature of the insomnia complaint. Drugs with a rapid absorption rate are better suited for sleep-onset insomnia, whereas those with a slower action are more effective for sleep-maintenance problems.

Flurazepam (Dalmane) is a rapidly absorbed hypnotic with an active metabolite that is slowly eliminated. Because the dosage interval is smaller than the half-life, there is a corresponding accumulation with nightly use. After termination of dosage, washout of active substances is correspondingly slow. Flurazepam is effective in both inducing and maintaining sleep for up to 1 month of consecutive nightly administration (A. Kales, Soldatos, & Vela-Bueno, 1985; Mitler, Seidel, Van Den Hoed, Greenblatt, & Dement, 1984; Bliwise, Seidel, Greenblatt, & Dement, 1984; Roehrs, Zorick, Kaffeman, Sickelsteel, & Roth, 1982).

Temazepam (Restoril) is a benzodiazepine with an intermediate half-life, which produces a moderate degree of accumulation with multiple dosage. It has a relatively slow rate of absorption and is a better agent for sleep-maintenance than for sleep-onset problems (Bixler, Kales, Soldatos, Scharf, & Kales, 1978; Mitler et al., 1979; Nicholson & Stone, 1979b; Roehrs, Lamphere, et al., 1984). For equal hypnotic effect, temazepam may produce the least residual impairment, and minimal tolerance has been reported for up to 3 months of use (Allen, Mendels, Nevins, Chernik, &

Hoddes, 1987). Because it is better suited for sleep-maintenance difficulties and has minimal daytime residual effects, temazepam is probably the best hypnotic to use for late-life insomnia (Morin, Stone, et al., 1993).

Triazolam (Halcion) has a fast absorption rate and a very short elimination half-life, such that minimal accumulation occurs during multiple-dose treatment. Its efficacy in reducing sleep-onset latency and increasing total sleep time is well documented (Mitler et al., 1984; Roth, Hartse, Saab, Piccione, & Kramer, 1980; Mamelak, Csima, & Price, 1984). Compared with the long-half-life hypnotics, triazolam produces less daytime sleepiness. However, early-morning awakening and daytime anxiety have been associated with this agent (Adam & Oswald, 1989; Carskadon, Seidel, Greenblatt, & Dement, 1982; A. Kales, Soldatos, Bixler, & Kales, 1983).

Estazolam (ProSom) and quazepam (Doral) are the two benzodiazepine hypnotics most recently approved by the FDA. Estazolam has a rapid onset of action and a moderate elimination half-life. Clinical studies indicate that it may remain effective for up to 6 weeks of nightly administration, though the average reduction of sleep-onset latency is a modest 15–20 minutes (Pierce & Shu, 1990). Quazepam has a pharmacokinetic profile similar to that of flurazepam, and is effective for the management of sleep-onset and sleep-maintenance insomnia (A. Kales et al., 1982; Mamelak et al., 1984). It produces less impairment of daytime functioning than flurazepam (Dement, 1991b), and its long half-life minimizes rebound insomnia.

Various benzodiazepine anxiolytics are frequently prescribed for insomnia associated with anxiety disorders. However, there is limited empirical evidence supporting the efficacy of medications such as diazepam (Valium), alprazolam (Xanax), lorazepam (Ativan), or oxazepam (Serax) as effective methods for treating insomnia. All benzodiazepines have anxiolytic, sedative–hypnotic, and anticonvulsant properties in ascending order of dose and brain concentration (Greenblatt & Shader, 1985; Poling, Gadow, & Cleary, 1991). Accordingly, anxiety is often relieved with doses that do not cause somnolence. With higher dosage, these drugs may achieve excellent anxiolytic and sedative effects, but they may also cause residual sedation that impairs daytime performance and alertness.

## Nonbenzodiazepine Hypnotics

Several nonbenzodiazepine hypnotics are currently under development for FDA approval or are already approved for use in countries other than the United States. Zolpidem is a hypnotic of rapid onset and short duration. It has been found effective in decreasing sleep-onset latency, but not in decreasing either the number or duration of awakenings. Therapeutic gains are well maintained for 5 weeks and slow-wave sleep is relatively well preserved. As for most short-acting hypnotics, there is evidence of rebound insomnia upon withdrawal from Zolpidem (Kryger, Steljes, Pouliot, Neufeld, & Odynski, 1991; Vogel, Scharf, Walsh, & Roth, 1989). Zopiclone, also a nonbenzodiazepine hypnotic, is rapidly absorbed (30 minutes to 1.5 hours), and its elimination half-life is about 6 hours. Several clinical trials in Canada and in France have shown that it is an effective agent for sleep-onset insomnia, and it produces less residual daytime anxiety (Fontaine, Beaudry, Le Morvan, Beauclair, & Chouinard, 1990) or rebound insomnia (Fleming, McClure, Mayes, Phillips, & Bourgouin, 1990) than a shorter-acting drug such as triazolam. Zopiclone has also produced significant decrease in anxiety symptoms among insomniacs with generalized anxiety disorder (Fontaine et al., 1990).

## Antidepressants

Tricyclic antidepressants with sedative effects are usually recommended when insomnia is associated with an affective disorder (A. Kales & Kales, 1984; Ware, 1983). This is probably a better choice than benzodiazepines, especially among patients with suicidal risk. Amitriptyline (Elavil) and trimipramine (Surmontil) reduce sleep-onset latency and improve sleep continuity (Shipley et al., 1985; Ware, Brown, Moorad, Pitlard, & Cobert, 1989). Trazodone (Desyrel), a nontricyclic, is increasingly used for insomnia in depressed patients (Goldberg & Finnerty, 1980). This compound may increase slow-wave sleep, and it appears to have less anticholinergic action and fewer cardiovascular side effects than tricyclics. As a general rule, insomniacs with major depression should receive the entire dosage of antidepressant at bedtime in order to maximize the sedative effects.

There is an increasing trend among physicians to prescribe anti-depressant medications rather than benzodiazepines for treating insomnia even in nondepressed individuals. Because of their sedating properties, some antidepressants are prescribed in subtherapeutic dosage (e.g., 10–20 milligrams of Elavil or Sinequan). Although the potential for abuse or physical dependency is lower with these agents, there is a higher potential for drug interaction than with benzodiazepines. Also, more energizing antidepressants may actually worsen sleep difficulties (protriptyline, fluoxetine) and should not be used for insomnia. Whereas the REM-suppressing effects of anti-depressants are well documented among patients with major depression (Reynolds & Kupfer, 1987; Rush et al., 1986), there has been no empirical study documenting their effects on the sleep of nondepressed insomniacs.

## Over-the-Counter Sleep Aids

Over-the-counter sleep aids are probably used in greater proportions than prescribed hypnotics. The active ingredient in most of them is an antihistamine, and because the most common side effect of antihistamines is drowsiness, people use them to promote sleep at night. Most antihistamines produce few beneficial effects on sleep, however. Despite a wide variety of over-the-counter sleeping medications (e.g., Sominex, Unisom, Sleep-Eze), these highly advertised drugs have received very little research attention, and their impact on sleep beyond a placebo effect is doubtful (Balter & Uhlenhuth, 1991; J. D. Kales et al., 1971). Although one study showed that two aspirins at bedtime had some beneficial effects on sleep-maintenance variables (Hauri & Silberfarb, 1980), for the most part there is no evidence that over-the-counter remedies improve objective sleep parameters.

## Limitations and Daytime Residual Effects

Although most hypnotics are efficacious with short-term use, several limitations must be considered. Most importantly, few data are available on their long-term efficacy. Controlled drug trials are usually of short duration (1–6 weeks), and follow-ups are typically limited to evaluating withdrawal effects from 1 to 7 days after drug discontinuation. In addition, several problems are likely to arise either during the course of treatment or after its discontinuation: alteration of sleep stages, daytime residual effects, rebound insomnia, and dependence.

Most hypnotics alter the sleep architecture (i.e., the proportion of time spent in each sleep stage). Although efficiency, continuity, and duration of sleep are improved, sleep quality is often diminished. For example, almost all benzodiazepines increase stage 2 sleep, but at the same time they decrease the amount of stages 3–4 sleep, which is considered the most restorative sleep. Some compounds also diminish REM sleep, though this effect depends on dosage and varies across medications. Furthermore, benzodiazepine-induced EEG changes do not necessarily correspond to subjective perceptions of sleep quality (Church & Johnson, 1979; Schneider-Helmert, 1985, 1988).

Daytime sedation, cognitive and psychomotor impairment, and drug "hangover" are all adverse side effects that must be weighed against the initial sleep benefits obtained from pharmacotherapy. Long-acting drugs produce more daytime sleepiness and greater impairment of waking performance than do short-acting ones (Dement, Seidel, & Carskadon, 1982; Johnson & Chernik, 1982; Roth & Roehrs, 1991). Elderly patients using long-acting drugs are at greater risks for falls and hip fractures than those using short-acting medications or no medication at all. Hypnotics with rapid elimination have been implicated in the production of anterograde amnesia; this appears to be a more serious problem, particularly with triazolam when used in a large dose (0.5 milligram) (Roth et al., 1980; Spinweber & Johnson, 1982). Whether the amnesia is attributable to the drug or to a state-dependent learning factor is unclear. Nevertheless, triazolam has been withdrawn from the market in several European countries. Overall, there is little empirical evidence, if any, to suggest that the performance decrements attributable to hypnotic use are compensated for by improved sleep.

Tolerance is an important shortcoming of drug therapy. Although tolerance varies across individuals, most drugs lose their effectiveness when used on a nightly basis. Larger doses are then required to achieve any effect, and when the highest dosage is reached, the patient is caught in a dead-end situation. Rebound insomnia, an intense worsening of sleep relative to baseline levels, is common after the drug is discontinued; this is particularly pronounced with short-acting drugs (Gillin et al., 1989; Roehrs, Vogel, & Roth, 1990). As much as a 60% increase in total wake time above baseline level has been reported on the first night following discontinuation of triazolam (A. Kales et al., 1985). This rebound is often accompanied by severe anxiety. With longer-acting drugs, the withdrawal effects are not as marked and develop only days after sleep medication is discontinued, but typically last longer. In any case, this rebound phenomenon tends to reinforce insomniacs' belief that they cannot sleep without medication. As such, it is extremely powerful in prompting patients to resume medication use and in promoting drug dependency.

## Indications and Contraindications

There are several clinical situations in which a short-term trial on a sleep-promoting medication can be helpful (Gillin & Byerley, 1990; NIH, 1984; Roth, Zorick, Wittig, & Roehrs, 1982). For example, it may be indicated in cases of acute insomnia resulting from situational stressors (e.g., death of a loved one, impending surgery). Short-term use of hypnotics may also be indicated for jet lag. Moreover, it may be appropriate when severe insomnia is attributable to an underlying sleep disorder (restless legs or periodic leg movements), an acute medical condition (pain), or selected psychiatric disorders. For persistent psychophysiological insomnia, hypnotic drugs should be considered adjuncts to the main therapeutic endeavor directed toward the perpetuating factors. Such symptomatic treatment can be particularly useful in the initial intervention phase for breaking the vicious cycle of insomnia, emotional arousal, and more sleep disturbances (Morin & Kwentus, 1988). After completion of a behavioral treatment program, the sole availability of a sleeping aid may minimize the risks of relapse. Drug therapy alone, however, is usually not successful for treating chronic insomnia. The only two comparative studies of behavioral and pharmacological therapies indicate that whereas pharmacotherapy may produce quicker results, clinical benefits are better maintained over time in those receiving behavior therapy either alone or in combination with drugs (McClusky, Milby, Switzer, Williams, & Wooten, 1991; Morin, Stone, et al., 1993). In any circumstance, medication should be used only for a short duration and should not exceed more than two doses per week, in order to avoid habituation (NIH, 1984).

Benzodiazepines are contraindicated in pregnant women, substance abusers, sleep apnea patients, and people who may unexpectedly be called on duties in the middle of the night. Although some hypnotics may be helpful in patients with generalized anxiety disorder (Fontaine et al., 1990), they should not be used in those with major depression who are at suicidal risk. As a general rule, insomnia associated with major psychopathology is best managed by treating the underlying disorder (antidepressants in depression, neuroleptics in psychosis, etc.). Clinical use of hypnotics in the geriatric population warrants special caution (Moran, Thompson, Nies, & Alan, 1988; NIH, 1991; Prinz, Vitiello, Raskind, & Thorpy, 1990). Older adults are more sensitive to drugs and metabolize them more slowly than younger people. Accordingly, elderly patients respond to smaller doses than younger subjects, and they are especially at risk for toxic effects of drugs with a long half-life. Long-acting drugs can create nocturnal confusion, can result in cognitive and motor impairment, and can increase the risks of falls in older patients, as noted above. Daytime carryover effects, such as sleepiness and reduced alertness, are also more pronounced in the medicated elderly (Kramer & Schoen, 1984). Multiple-drug interactions and noncompliance with the prescribed regimen represent additional potential problems, not only with the elderly but with all hypnotic users.

In sum, hypnotic medications are efficacious on a short-term basis, but there are few data available on their efficacy with prolonged use. They can be useful adjuncts in the treatment of insomnia but should be used cautiously. Their initial clinical benefits must be weighed against their daytime sequelae and long-term effects. When pharmacotherapy is initiated, there is always a danger of prolonged use, despite the initial intent of relying on the medication only for a limited duration. Moreover, regardless of the medication subtype, prolonged use of sleep aids undermines the development of appropriate self-management skills and coping strategies. From a psychological perspective, the use of sleep medications in chronic insomnia is likely to reinforce the perception that one is a victim of insomnia and as such has no control over sleep.

## A Program for Withdrawal from Sleep Medications

### Prevalence and Natural History of Drug Dependency

The NIMH survey of psychotherapeutic drug use reported that 7.1% of adults have used either a prescribed or an over-the-counter sleep aid in the course of a year, and that 11% of hypnotic users had used their medication regularly for a year or longer (Mellinger et al., 1985). Among patients seeking treatment at our insomnia clinic, about 80% present with a current or past history of usage of sleep aids, and 50–60% are habitual drug users in that they consume sleep aids two nights or more per week. Older adults and women are more likely to consume sleep medications (Morgan et al., 1988), as are those with higher psychological distress (Mellinger et al., 1985).

Drug-taking behaviors can follow several patterns. Drug-dependent insomnia involves nearly daily use of a hypnotic for 3 weeks or more; by definition, it also implies tolerance to or withdrawal from hypnotic medications (ASDA, 1990). In contrast, prolonged users remain on normal therapeutic doses for extensive periods of time without evidence of tolerance (Mendelson, 1980). Other individuals are habitual users who limit their medication intake to two or three nights per week. Although self-contained, this pattern of use may still be chronic, in that some have been using medications for several months and sometimes years. The types of drug-taking behaviors discussed here are not limited to prescribed medications, for a substantial number of insomniacs also self-medicate with alcohol, over-the-counter medications, and/or recreational drugs.

Abuse or misuse of prescribed medications has received little attention, in comparison to abuse/misuse of alcohol and recreational drugs (Roy-Byrne & Cowley, 1991). Although the potential for benzodiazepine abuse is lower than that for abuse of other substances, drug-dependent insomnia is a significant clinical problem. This dependency, which is analogous to drug dependency among anxious patients, is often more psychological than physical in nature. It rarely develops overnight; rather, it evolves in a gradual fashion (i.e., use, tolerance, withdrawal, and dependence). Patients are typically introduced to hypnotics during periods of acute stress, during hospitalization, or at times when they can no longer cope with chronic insomnia. Prescriptions are sometimes renewed automatically, even though the insomnia may have subsided. Close monitoring is not always conducted, and patients often exceed recommended guidelines. Tolerance may develop with nightly use, so that increased dosage is required to achieve any hypnotic effects. When the maximum safe dosage has been reached, the patient is trapped in a dead-end situation. Therapeutic dosage no longer works, yet any attempt to discontinue the medication is followed by worsening of sleep difficulties above and beyond baseline levels. The patient re-enters a cycle of catastrophic thinking and misinterpretations of insomnia symptoms. The lack of information about the transient nature of these withdrawal effects often leads to excessive concerns and return to medication. The belief that medication is indeed necessary is reinforced, and the vicious cycle is perpetuated. As several studies have shown, attributional processes play an important role in perpetuating medication use (Bootzin, Herman, & Nicassio, 1976; Davidson, Tsujimoto, & Glaros, 1973; Storms & Nisbett, 1970). Thus, both the lack of standard monitoring procedures and the absence of patient education may contribute to prolonged use of sleep medications.

Conditioning principles also play an important role in perpetuating the compulsive use of hypnotics. Insomnia and its sequelae can be conceptualized as an aversive state. The hypnotic and anxiolytic properties of most benzodiazepines terminate this aversive state, and the drug-taking behavior is negatively reinforced. To maintain effectiveness and prevent tolerance, intermittent use (i.e., "as needed") is the schedule of choice. However, this intermittent schedule is also quite powerful in perpetuating a self-contained yet habitual pattern of use. As such, it creates a vicious cycle (insomnia, medication intake, tolerance, cessation of medication, rebound insomnia, resumption of medication, etc; see Figure 11.1).

According to classical conditioning principles, repeated pairings of hypnotic medications (unconditioned stimulus) with falling asleep (unconditioned response) should theoretically lead to a conditioned sleep response in the absence of medication. However, the phenomenon of conditioned tolerance takes precedence over this. Animal studies indicate that the conditoned response is often opposite or antagonistic to the direct effect of the drug (Siegel, 1983). For example, morphine produces analgesia, but the con-

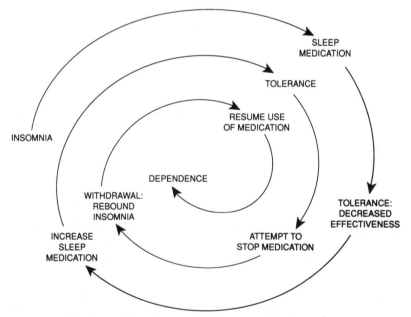

**FIGURE 11.1.** The vicious cycle of drug-dependent insomnia.

ditioned response elicited by environmental cues associated with its previous administration is hyperalgesia, an increase in pain sensitivity. A similar phenomenon occurs with the sedative actions of benzodiazepines (King et al., 1987). Animals receiving repeated dosages of benzodiazepines in the same environment are more tolerant to the drugs than those receiving them in a different setting. Subsequent exposure to the same situational context can then precipitate withdrawal symptoms in the absence of the drugs. In chronic insomniacs, hypnotic use is associated with temporal (bedtime) and environmental (bed/bedroom) stimuli. With repeated use, the antagonistic conditioned response elicited by those cues grows progressively stronger and diminishes the effect of the drug. Tolerance is then enhanced, and when the medication is discontinued, symptoms of withdrawal are more pronounced. However, as previously stated, intermittent use minimizes tolerance. Thus, when hypnotic medications are used on an "as-needed" basis, which is similar to an intermittent reinforcement schedule, extinction of the drug-taking behavior is correspondingly slow.

Misperception of sleep–wake patterns also plays a leading role in a patient's inability to escape sleeping pills. It is well known that drug-free insomniacs overestimate sleep-onset latency and underestimate total sleep time relative to EEG criteria (Carskadon et al., 1976; Coates et al., 1982). In medicated insomniacs, however, there is a reverse trend in that they overestimate hypnotic efficacy. Schneider-Helmert (1988) found that his patients overestimated sleep duration by 72 minutes relative to EEG recordings while on medication. In contrast, under withdrawal conditions they overestimated sleep-onset latency by 1 hour. Thus, the subjective perception of sleep is impaired in medicated insomniacs. They have a reduced recollection of wakefulness while on medication and become acutely aware of their sleep disturbances upon withdrawal. Anterograde amnesia, a well-established side effect of some benzodiazepines, is the most likely explanation of this phenomenon. These memory impairments produce perceptual distortions of sleep–wake patterns, which in turn strengthen patients' attributions of improved sleep to medication effects. These findings are even more intriguing when we consider that the sleep architecture of medicated insomniacs is objectively more disturbed than that of insomniacs who are unmedicated. For instance, the proportions of stages 3–4 and REM sleep are significantly lower in medicated subjects (Schneider-Helmert, 1988), and these individuals show sleep difficulty as severe as that of drug-free insomniacs even when they are using drugs.

In summary, several factors combine to perpetuate use of sleep medications and insomnia: the lack of standard monitoring procedures, the absence of patient education, the powerful effect of intermittent hypnotic use, conditioned tolerance, and misperceptions of sleep–wake patterns when medicated. Some as-yet-unidentified personality variables may also predispose some individuals to hypnotic abuse and dependence. A structured withdrawal program is outlined in the remainder of this section, along with clinical guidelines to facilitate its implementation.

## Assessment of Drug Use Pattern

The clinician should already have obtained during the initial evaluation a comprehensive drug history, including the types of sleeping aids (both prescribed and over-the-counter), as well as the dosage, frequency of use, and duration of usage. Current pattern of use should be based on two time periods: a retrospective report for 1 month preceding the initial visit, and at least 2 weeks of prospective baseline daily monitoring. These two assessments may yield different patterns of use. Some patients minimize their drug use during the initial evaluation; others are reactive to self-monitoring and temporarily decrease medication during baseline assessment.

## Setting Goals

An example of a weekly monitoring form, with entries for types of sleep aids, dosage, and frequency of use, is presented in Table 11.2. Once baseline values are established, weekly goals for targeted dosage and number of medicated nights should be set. A self-efficacy rating reflecting the patient's confidence in achieving his or her goals is obtained. It is preferable to set gradual and attainable goals for which the patient expresses a high level of self-confidence. In the latter part of the withdrawal schedule, drug-free nights are predetermined ahead of time. Outcome is measured by the number of medicated nights and by the percentage of dosage reduction.

Before implementing this treatment component, the clinician should re-examine the patient's attitudes toward drug treatments and readiness to discontinue medication. Motivations for getting off medication should also be explored. Outcome can be affected by whether the motivation is extrinsic (e.g., pressure from a spouse) rather than intrinsic (e.g., a desire to achieve more self-control). Furthermore, though being entirely drug-free is ideal, it may not be realistic or desirable for patients who are under severe stress (e.g., divorce) and those presenting with acute pain. Because of the potential risks associated with withdrawal from sedative–hypnotics, it is essential to enlist the collaboration of a physician or a pharmacist, especially in the initial planning phase. Ideally, this should involve the patient's prescribing physician.

TABLE 11.2. A Sample Medication Withdrawal Schedule

| Week | Type | Dosage (mg) | No. of nights Actual | No. of nights Target | Total amount (mg) | % dosage reduction | Self-efficacy (0–100%) |
|---|---|---|---|---|---|---|---|
| Interview | ProSom | 2 | 7 | — | 14 | — | — |
| Week 1 | ProSom | 2 | 5 | — | 10 | — | — |
| Week 2 | ProSom | 2 | 7 | — | 14 | — | — |
| Week 3 | ProSom | 1 | 7 | 7 | 7 | 50% | 80% |
| Week 4 | ProSom | 1 | 6 | 5 | 6 | 57% | 65% |
| Week 5 | ProSom | 1 | 5 | 5 | 5 | 64% | 75% |
| Week 6 | ProSom | 1 | 4 | 4 | 4 | 71% | 80% |
| Week 7 | ProSom | 1 | 4 | 3 | 4 | 71% | 75% |
| Week 8 | ProSom | 1 | 3 | 2 | 3 | 79% | 60% |
| Week 9 | ProSom | 1 | 1 | 1 | 1 | 93% | 80% |
| Week 10 | ProSom | 1 | 0 | 0 | 0 | 100% | 75% |

## Education

Providing factual information about the short- and long-term effects of drugs on sleep is an integral part of this withdrawal program. Using a didactic approach, the clinician should explain the effects of benzodiazepines on duration, continuity, and quality of sleep in lay terms. The effects of the specific agent used by the patient should be discussed. For example, a patient with sleep-onset difficulties who is using temazepam may be interested to know that this is not the best choice of medication, as it has a relatively slow onset of action and is more appropriate for sleep-maintenance problems. Triazolam may be ideal for delayed sleep onset, but its short-acting properties may subsequently cause early morning awakening (A. Kales, Soldatos, et al., 1983). Issues of habituation and dependence should be discussed, and a conceptual framework explaining the nature of the vicious cycle in which the patient is caught should be provided (see Figure 11.1). Limitations and side effects should also be reviewed, and any misconceptions the patient may have should be corrected. Several long-acting drugs, as noted above, carry daytime residual effects (e.g., impaired alertness and performance); these deficits are often mistakenly attributed to disturbed sleep.

Potential withdrawal effects associated with discontinuation of benzo-diazepines may include rebound insomnia, anxiety, irritability, fatigue, headache, muscle tremors, nausea, and increased perceptual acuity (Roy-Byrne & Hommer, 1988). These effects vary according to the specific agent used, its dosage, and its half-life. Intensity of withdrawal symptoms is more severe with short-acting drugs, particularly if such drugs are abruptly discontinued. Although some of these effects may be pseudowithdrawal effects resulting from expectations of re-emerging distressing symptoms, they should still be monitored carefully.

It is important to prepare the patient for the potential adverse symptoms that may be experienced as the medication is discontinued. For example, rebound insomnia and daytime anxiety are common upon discontinuation of rapidly eliminated hypnotics, as noted earlier (Adam & Oswald, 1989; Gillin et al., 1989). The patient should be informed of the transient nature of these withdrawal effects. This will prevent catastrophic interpretation that chronic insomnia has returned, and minimize reinforcement of the underlying belief that medication is indeed necessary. This didactic component is not intended to scare the patient unduly or to induce apprehension about the ill effects of sleep medication. The main objectives are to inform the consumer, promote adaptive cognitions, enhance motivation and compliance with the medication withdrawal regimen, and prepare the patient for potential rebound effects.

## Withdrawal Schedules

Current standards of clinical practice suggest that a patient should be tapered off a sedative–hypnotic at the rate of one therapeutic dose per week. Specific withdrawal schedules should be individualized according to the type, dosage, frequency, and duration of drug use.

The first step in the tapering-off process is to stabilize the patient on the lowest available dosage of the drug in question. For example, a nightly dosage of 30 milligrams of flurazepam would initially be reduced to 15 milligrams per night. When several drugs are combined or alternated, the patient should first be stabilized on a single medication. When the highest recommended dosage is used intermittently (i.e., three to four nights per week), a useful strategy is to reduce the initial dosage and allow the patient to use the medication every night. This process should take 1 to 2 weeks, depending on the number and dosage of the sleeping aids involved. Use of a gradual withdrawal schedule is preferable to abrupt discontinuation because it minimizes rebound effects (Greenblatt, Harmatz, Zinny, & Shader, 1987). It is also more acceptable to those patients who initially display high anxiety levels. Switching from a short- to a long-acting compound that has built-in tapering action may also minimize rebound effects. This is clinically important, because rebound effects are often what perpetuate use of sleep medications in patients who may otherwise wish to discontinue their usage.

Several problems may arise when the lowest available dosage has been reached. The smallest available dosages are 15 milligrams for flurazepam, 7.5 milligrams for temazepam, and 0.125 milligram for triazolam. Although some medications are sold in tablets and can be split in half, others are available only in gelatin capsules, which makes the task cumbersome. Liquid equivalents may be used on an inpatient basis but are impractical in an outpatient context. An equally difficult task is to design an effective schedule for individuals using medication at its lowest available dose on an "as-needed" basis. Most insomniacs are well aware of the contraindications to using medications every night, and often limit their use to two or three nights per week. This intermittent use minimizes tolerance and maintains effectiveness for longer periods of time; however, as noted earlier, this schedule also prolongs reliance on medication and promotes dependency. Several additional guidelines can facilitate the withdrawal process at this stage.

Once stabilization on the smallest dosage has been reached, the next step consists of introducing drug-free nights. Medication is allowed only on a number of predetermined nights. Depending on the frequency of use, this may entail skipping one night the first week, two nights the second, and so on. It is best to skip medications first on weekend nights. Intermittent users consume hypnotics on the nights preceding demanding days when important tasks or events are scheduled. They want to ensure a good night's sleep in order to maintain adequate daytime functioning. There are usually fewer occupational obligations on weekends, and apprehensions of impairments on these days should also be lower. "Drug holidays" are then introduced on weeknights. A similar rationale is followed, in that nights preceding less demanding days are preselected.

The next rule consists of making medication use time-contingent rather than insomnia-contingent. The patient is instructed to take his or her usual drug on preselected nights and at a fixed time (i.e., 30 minutes before bedtime), regardless of whether or not sleeplessness is expected. Although this may initially lead to increased usage, particularly when the patient believes he or she might not need the drug, this method is helpful to weaken the association between sleeplessness and drug-taking behavior.

Except for the fact that a gradual schedule is preferable to an abrupt one, little research has compared the efficacy of various hypnotic withdrawal schedules. The pain literature, however, suggests that delivery of narcotics at fixed intervals is superior to an "as-needed" schedule, both for decreasing pain ratings and for reducing medication intake (Berntzen & Gotestam, 1987; White & Sanders, 1985).

## Timing of Medication Withdrawal

Should insomniacs be tapered off their medications before, during, or after implementation of the psychological management program? In an elegant study addressing this issue, Espie, Lindsay, and Brooks (1988) compared two protocols in which five chronic hypnotic users were withdrawn before and five after receiving behavioral therapies. The patients who were first withdrawn from medication achieved better outcome on sleep-onset latency than those withdrawn after behavioral treatment. Assignment to these conditions was strictly based on each patient's choice, and the most severely insomniac patients tended to choose the late withdrawal program. Thus, initial insomnia severity and anxiety levels are important factors in determining the timing of the medication withdrawal.

Prospective subjects in outcome research are typically required to discontinue hypnotic use prior to entering a given treatment protocol. Although this requirement minimizes confounding effects, it also greatly limits generalization of the findings. Patients with the most severe insomnia are often unable or simply unwilling to discontinue their medications unless an alternative treatment is concurrently available. These individuals are the ones most likely to seek nonpharmacological therapies. Accordingly, it seems preferable to integrate the medication withdrawal plan within the overall clinical protocol.

The relative efficacy of a medication withdrawal plan implemented in the context of a brief consultation or as part of a comprehensive stress management program was evaluated with drug-dependent insomniacs (Kirmil-Gray, Eagleston, Thoresen, & Zarcone, 1985). Both interventions successfully eliminated medication use in an average duration of 8 weeks. Although sleep improvements were modest at posttreatment, possibly because of persisting rebound effects, subjects receiving concurrent stress management showed greater improvements of sleep and mood compared to those receiving a brief consultation focused exclusively on medication withdrawal. These results are consistent with findings obtained in anxious patients, in whom withdrawal effects are minimized when the medication reduction plan is combined with cognitive-behavioral therapy (Sanchez-Craig, Kay, Busto, & Cappell, 1986). One recent controlled evaluation of relaxation therapy for geriatric insomnia found this intervention effective for decreasing hypnotic usage among older adults (Lichstein & Johnson, 1993).

A psychological intervention implemented concurrently with a structured medication withdrawal plan should facilitate elimination of sleep aids. The sole discontinuation of hypnotics may improve sleep in some insomniacs. More frequently, however, residual sleep disturbances often persist even after complete drug elimination, and additional treatment is often needed. Some individuals are also too anxious about stopping their medication early in the program. With these people, it is preferable to introduce this component only after they have been exposed to the cognitive-behavioral procedures, so that they have something to fall back on to help cope with residual sleep disturbances.

## Summary of Clinical Guidelines

Successful withdrawal from sleep medication depends upon a number of factors, including prior drug use pattern, insomnia severity, specific withdrawal schedules, and patient characteristics. These factors should dictate the optimal timing for introducing a given withdrawal plan, as well as its duration. Complete elimination of hypnotic use is facilitated when the withdrawal program is judiciously integrated with cognitive-behavioral strategies.

1. A structured program is essential. Simply encouraging patients to reduce medication is unlikely to be successful. Studies with long-term users of benzodiazepines, primarily anxious patients, have shown that a formal withdrawal plan is essential to decreasing consumption of anxiolytics (Fraser, Peterkin, Gamsu, & Baldwin, 1990). Whether the program is implemented by a general medical practitioner or a mental health professional does not affect outcome, as long as it includes a specified withdrawal schedule. Close monitoring and regular follow-ups are essential to prevent relapse.

2. Education and support should be integral elements of any sleep medication withdrawal program. Many patients who are apparently too anxious to discontinue medication are never given an opportunity to try an alternative intervention. The clinician needs to teach these individuals that long-term use is unnecessary and that withdrawal effects are time-limited. It is also essential to convey a sense that they can learn coping skills to replace the anxiolytic–hypnotic effects formerly provided by their drugs.

3. Patients' motivation and compliance are equally important factors. The desire to achieve better self-control over sleep is one of the most important motivations for seeking treatment. To enhance this perception of self-control, each patient should be allowed to decide when the withdrawal schedule is to be introduced, on which night dosage is to be reduced, and which nights are to be drug-free. The clinician needs to provide structure, yet the specific withdrawal protocol needs to be patient-driven.

4. Specific withdrawal schedules should be individualized according to the type, dosage, frequency, and duration of drug use. A gradual withdrawal is preferable to abrupt discontinuation. Patients eager to stop their medications should be advised to avoid doing so abruptly, as this may enhance the potential for withdrawal effects and perpetuate reliance on medications.

5. The collaboration of a physician or pharmacist is essential in designing a safe withdrawal schedule. It may even be necessary to admit heavy users

to a hospital for a closely supervised inpatient detoxication program. This is occasionally the case for older patients who have been using large doses of barbiturates and not only have become dependent but are experiencing severe toxic effects. In most cases, however, the drug dependency is relatively self-contained, and the patients seek alternative therapies because they wish to achieve better self-control or because the drug simply is no longer working. As such, the program outlined here is more likely to be effective for insomniacs who have developed iatrogenic dependency than for those who are actively abusing sedative–hypnotics.

# III

## CLINICAL EFFICACY

# 12

## Treatment Outcome Evaluations

This last chapter reviews empirical findings from two large data sets of outcome evaluations. The first section summarizes the results of a clinical replication series involving 100 insomnia patients treated in our clinic over the past 5 years with the treatment protocol described in this book. The second section presents the results of a meta-analysis of 59 outcome studies evaluating the clinical efficacy of more than a dozen different psychological interventions for insomnia. I conclude by discussing the impact of several moderating variables (e.g., patients' characteristics, treatment modality, contextual factors) on treatment efficacy.

### Clinical Replication Series

The majority of insomnia outcome studies have used community-recruited subjects to evaluate treatment effects. Very few have been based on patients spontaneously seeking treatment (Edinger & Stout, 1985) or on those referred by physicians (Espie, Lindsay, Brooks, et al., 1989; Sanavio et al., 1990). It is unclear whether unsolicited insomniacs present with the same sleep problem severity and respond to treatment to the same extent as those specifically recruited from the community for participation in clinical trials. This is an important issue, because only a small proportion of insomnia sufferers seek treatment (Mellinger et al., 1985), and these individuals tend to display more psychological distress than those who participate in outcome research (Stepanski et al., 1989). In addition, most controlled evaluations have typically excluded individuals whose insomnia is complicated by hypnotic use, psychopathology, or chronic medical illnesses; this has limited the generalizibility of research findings. These special populations are probably at greater risk of developing sleep disturbances, and certainly those most in need of non-pharmacological treatment.

Over the past several years, my colleagues and I have evaluated the clinical efficacy of the treatment protocol described in this manual with a heterogeneous group of insomniacs presenting to our clinic (Morin, Stone, et al., 1992). In this section, I describe the clinical characteristics of this sample and summarize the treatment findings. It is important to note that the data did not come from a controlled trial; rather, they were gathered as part of a clinical replication series. As such, these outcome findings reflect more adequately the type of results to expect with patients typically seen in clinical practice. The only criteria for inclusion in this case series were that patients had to present with a chief complaint of insomnia, that they had to attend a minimum of three sessions, and that sleep diary data had to be available for at least 1 week of baseline and 2 weeks of treatment. Of more than 200 consecutive patients evaluated for insomnia in our sleep disorders clinic, we retained 100 patients who met those criteria. The remaining patients were either not interested in treatment or presented with a concomitant disorder deemed to require separate and prior intervention (e.g., major depression, substance abuse). Some patients were also excluded from this case series because their insomnia was associated with other sleep disorders (e.g., sleep apnea, periodic limb movements, circadian disorders). People who were unable to keep a sleep diary because of severe psychopathology (e.g., psychosis) or cognitive impairments (e.g., dementia) were treated, but no data are available to document their treatment response.

## Demographic and Clinical Characteristics

The 100 patients were 64 women and 36 men with an average age of 45 years ($SD = 13.8$ years); 60% were married. Although their socioeconomic background varied extensively, the majority (69%) of patients were employed, and their education level averaged 14.9 years. The patients presented with a chief complaint of either sleep-onset ($n = 18$), sleep-maintenance ($n = 18$), or mixed ($n = 64$) insomnia. Their average insomnia duration was 10.7 years, and 84% had used a sleep aid at least once in the month preceding the initial evaluation.

As can be seen from Figure 12.1, the majority of patients (74%) met criteria for psychophysiological insomnia ($n = 31$), insomnia associated with psychopathology ($n = 22$), or drug-dependent insomnia ($n = 21$). The remaining patients received a primary diagnosis of insomnia secondary to medical disorders (mostly pain-related) ($n = 13$), idiopathic insomnia ($n = 8$), or adjustment sleep disorder ($n = 5$). Although the origins of insomnia varied extensively across individuals, more than 56% met criteria for psychophysiological insomnia as either a primary or secondary sleep diagnosis. Because nocturnal polysomnography was conducted on only a small proportion of patients, it is plausible that some of these patients had a primary diagnosis of subjective (i.e., sleep state misperception) rather than psy-

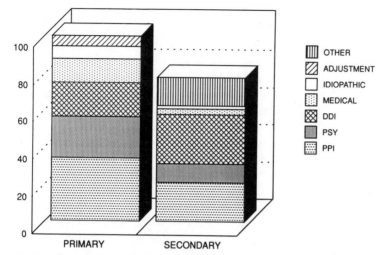

**FIGURE 12.1.** Sleep diagnoses in a series of 100 insomniacs. PPI, psychophysiological insomnia; PSY, insomnia associated with psychopathology; DDI, drug-dependent insomnia.

chophysiological insomnia, though these were likely to represent fewer than 10% of all patients in the case series.

## Procedures

All patients completed a standard assessment protocol as described in Chapter 5. After the initial appointment was scheduled, each patient was mailed a sleep questionnaire/symptom checklist, sleep diaries, and several psychometric measures. Thereafter, patients were seen for one or two evaluation sessions devoted to further assessment of the sleep complaint and to a detailed functional analysis of its controlling factors. Patients also underwent one or two nights of nocturnal polysomnography when this was clinically indicated, in order to rule out the presence of sleep apnea or periodic limb movements, or to evaluate the severity of sleep disturbances.

Treatment was provided on an individual basis. Its format was short-term, structured, and sleep-focused. Therapy sessions were held on a weekly basis initially, and biweekly once all treatment components had been introduced. The mean number of therapy sessions attended was 7.8 (range = 3–52) conducted over an average of 14.3 weeks. When concomitant psychological dysfunctions were present, these problems were addressed (if the patient still wanted them addressed) after the insomnia treatment protocol had been implemented. If these psychological dysfunctions were the predominant complaints, either subjects were referred elsewhere, or they were treated in our clinic but their data were not included in the present case series. For example, patients occasionally presented with an initial complaint of insomnia, but during the course of the evaluation it became clear that marital difficulties, substance abuse, or major affective disorders were the primary problems and should be the target of treatment.

The intervention was multifaceted. The behavior therapy component (i.e., stimulus control and sleep restriction) was usually introduced first, followed by the cognitive and educational treatment modules, respectively. This sequence was altered when it was clear that a given factor (e.g., excessive caffeine intake) was the primary insomnia cause. For drug-dependent insomnia, the medication withdrawal component was generally implemented concomitantly with the other therapy components. The specific withdrawal schedule was based on the type, dosage, and frequency of sleep medication used by each patient, as well as on the patient's readiness to discontinue hypnotic medications. The presence of concomitant psychological or medical disorders also dictated the appropriateness of discontinuing sleep medications. For example, when major depression was present, it was not clinically appropriate to withdraw these patients from their antidepressant medications, even though these might have been prescribed for insomnia symptoms. Likewise, most of the pain patients who were referred to our clinic for sleep disturbances were on a small dose (10–20 milligrams) of amitriptyline, which was prescribed for its presumed analgesic and sedative effects. We did not have the freedom to alter their medication regimen, and the intervention was restricted to the other three treatment components with those patients.

## Outcome Data

Figure 12.2 summarizes the changes in total wake time for all clinical patients combined and for the three subgroups presenting with the most common insomnia subtypes. Results from the total sample, regardless of diagnoses, show that treatment produced substantial reductions of total wake time from pretreatment (153 minutes) to posttreatment (84 minutes), for an overall improvement rate of 45%. The magnitude of improvement was very similar across measures of sleep induction and sleep maintenance. Significant reductions of sleep-onset latency (56 to 31 minutes), wake after sleep onset (52 to 30 minutes), and early-morning awakening (49 to 27 minutes) were obtained, with the absolute values of all three variables falling below or returning near the 30-minute cutoff criterion typically used to define insomnia.

There was a very modest gain in total sleep time (i.e., 25 minutes). This is not unusual, because most interventions (whether behavioral or pharmacological in nature) rarely produce significant increase in sleep duration.

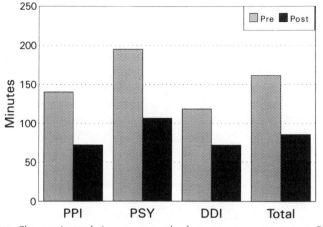

**FIGURE 12.2.** Changes in total time spent awake from pre- to posttreatment. PPI, psychophysiological insomnia; PSY, insomnia associated with psychopathology; DDI, drug-dependent insomnia.

Although many patients wish to increase their sleep time, this goal often needs to be adjusted, because total sleep time in insomniacs does not differ greatly from that in good sleepers to begin with. More often, it is sleep efficiency that is diminished, in that insomniacs need to spend more time in bed than noninsomniacs to achieve the same sleep duration. Thus, treatment is more effective in stabilizing sleep patterns and in consolidating sleep over a shorter period of time spent in bed. Sleep efficiency, rather than sleep duration alone, is probably a better index of sleep improvement, as it reflects one's abilities to initiate and maintain sleep relative to the amount of time spent in bed. Data on the distribution of sleep efficiency from pre- to posttreatment showed that 63 patients had a sleep efficiency of 80% or more after treatment, compared to only 25 patients prior to treatment. These results indicate that a fairly large number of patients moved from a dysfunctional to a functional range of sleep efficiency.

Patients whose insomnia was associated with psychopathology tended to have more severe sleep disruptions at baseline than did either psychophysiological or drug-dependent insomniacs. Although total sleep time was not significantly different across the three groups, psychopathology patients needed to spend significantly more time in bed to achieve comparable sleep durations; hence their lower sleep efficiency. In particular, problems with staying asleep were more severe in the psychopathology than in the drug-dependent insomnia group, perhaps owing to the fact that the latter group used medications more frequently. Nonetheless, despite using sleep medications on 90% of the nights, the drug-dependent insomniacs reported

as severe sleep disturbances at baseline as the psychophysiological insomniacs.

The pattern of changes on the various sleep variables was quite similar
across diagnostic groups. The absolute magnitude of changes was higher in
the psychopathology group, possibly because of some regression toward the
mean; in general, however, the amount of change on the various sleep
measures was fairly comparable across subgroups. For example, sleep efficiency improved significantly from pre- to posttreatment in all three groups
(as noted above), and the significant between-group differences in severity of
symptoms noted at baseline were no longer present at posttreatment.
Although significant sleep difficulties remained in the psychopathology
group, they were less severe than before treatment.

An important index of clinical improvement is the frequency with which
patients use sleep medications. The drug-dependent insomniacs achieved a
59% reduction of medication intake during the course of treatment, with 9 of
the initial 21 patients in this group being drug-free when they left the
program. Although this figure is far from an ideal outcome, it also indicates
that these patients were more confident in their self-management skills by the
time they left treatment. Only follow-up data will inform us of the durability
of this effect and of relapse rate over time. Although the psychophysiological
insomniacs were not classified as drug-dependent, significant reductions in
usage of sleep aids were obtained in this group as well. The number of
medicated nights went from two per week at baseline to less than one night
per week after treatment, and 22 subjects were drug-free after treatment,
compared to only 9 at baseline. The modest reduction of medication intake in
the psychopathology group is in part explained by the fact that it was not
always desirable or clinically indicated to decrease medication intake in this
patient population, as explained earlier.

In summary, these findings provide empirical evidence supporting the
use of cognitive-behavioral therapy for the management of insomnia across a
variety of patients. Improvement rates obtained for the main target symptoms
of sleep-onset latency and wake after sleep onset are fairly similar to those
obtained in controlled outcome evaluations (Lacks & Morin, 1992). The
findings also indicate that even though psychological treatment is not successful with all insomniacs, a substantial proportion can move from a dysfunctional to a functional range in terms of sleep efficiency. Although no data on
process–outcome relationships are available, clinical evidence suggests that
perception of control is an important element in the successful management
of insomnia. The patients who responded best to treatment also felt more in
control of their sleep, and reported that they could cope more adaptively with
residual and periodic sleep difficulties after treatment completion. Additional
mediating factors in treatment response are reviewed in a later section of this
chapter.

## Meta-Analytic Review of Outcome Studies

The discussion thus far has focused on the clinical efficacy of one multi-component intervention for insomnia. I now turn to the evaluation of each of the individual therapy components, as well as of several additional treatment methods used in the management of insomnia. Among these, relaxation-based treatments, biofeedback, and paradoxical intention have received the most empirical attention. Several literature reviews summarizing the benefits and limitations of these methods have been published in the past few years (Espie, 1991; Lacks & Morin, 1992; Lichstein & Fisher, 1985; Morin, 1991; Morin & Kwentus, 1988; Van Oot, Lane, & Borkovec, 1984).

The advent of meta-analytic procedures has greatly facilitated the systematic evaluation of treatment efficacy across multiple studies. In a meta-analysis, the effect size provides a standard metric for evaluating outcome across multiple studies. The effect size is used as a summary statistic to quantify treatment effectiveness and to examine the impact of moderating variables on outcome (treatment modality, patient characteristics, etc.).

My colleagues and I reviewed 59 controlled outcome studies comparing one or more psychological treatment methods for sleep-onset, sleep-maintenance, or mixed insomnia (Morin, Culbert, Kowatch, & Walton, 1989; Morin, Culbert, & Schwartz, 1993). These studies were identified through a computer search, bibliographies of previous reviews, and references of the studies themselves. Criteria for inclusion of a study in this meta-analysis were as follows: (1) The target problem was sleep-onset or sleep-maintenance insomnia; (2) the nature of treatment was nonpharmacological; (3) the study employed a group design; and (4) the outcome measures were sleep-onset latency, wake after sleep onset, number of awakenings, and/or total sleep time. Because of the paucity of studies using polysomnographic (i.e., EEG) measures, this meta-analysis was based on data collected from daily sleep diaries.

A total of 2,102 insomnia subjects were involved in the 59 studies selected. The majority of participants were recruited from the community, though a small minority were self-referred or physician-referred patients. Typical criteria for inclusion were that sleep-onset latency and/or wake after sleep onset exceeded 30 minutes on three or more nights per week, and that the insomnia problem had persisted for more than 6 months. The subjects were predominantly females (60%); they averaged 44 years of age, and reported a mean insomnia duration of 11 years.

Sleep-onset insomniacs took over 1 hour (65 minutes) to fall asleep at baseline, while those with sleep-maintenance insomnia reported an average of 70 minutes of wakefulness after sleep onset. Participants reported an average of two awakenings per night, with less than 6 hours of total sleep time per night. Most investigators selected individuals whose insomnia was pri-

behavioral and cognitive treatment modalities that target different facets of insomnia. There may also be some indications for integrating psychological and pharmacological approaches, though only two studies have thus far explored this biobehavioral option (McClusky et al., 1991; Morin, Stone, et al., 1993).

To make empirical research most relevant to clinical practice, we need to move beyond an exclusive focus on young, healthy, and drug-free individuals. We also need to broaden the scope of our interventions and to assess their impact on daytime functioning, psychological well-being, and the quality of life (Lacks & Morin, 1992). In sum, chronic insomnia is a complex and multifaceted problem that is difficult to treat. Effective treatment strategies are already available, but they need to be further refined to maximize therapeutic benefits and adapted to the needs of those most at risk for insomnia.

# APPENDICES

## APPENDIX A. Insomnia Interview Schedule

*Demographic Information*

Name:                                           Sex/race:
Address:                                        Age:
                                                Marital status:
                                                Occupation:
Phone:                                          Education:

1. *Nature of Sleep–Wake Problem*

| | | | | |
|---|---|---|---|---|
| Do you have a problem with falling asleep? | No | Mild | Moderate | Severe |
| Do you have a problem with staying asleep? | No | Mild | Moderate | Severe |
| Do you have a problem with waking up too early in the morning? | No | Mild | Moderate | Severe |
| Do you have a problem with staying awake during the day? | No | Mild | Moderate | Severe |

2. *Current Sleep–Wake Schedule*

| | |
|---|---|
| What is your usual bedtime on weekdays? | _____ o'clock |
| At what time do you last awaken in the morning? | _____ o'clock |
| What is your usual arising time on weekdays? | _____ o'clock |
| Do you have the same sleep–wake schedule on weekends? | Yes     No |
| How often do you take naps (including unintentional naps)? | _____ days/week |
| Do you ever fall asleep at inappropriate times/places? | Yes     No |
| How many nights/week do you have a problem with falling/staying asleep? | _____ nights |
| On a typical night (past month), how long does it take you to fall asleep after you go to bed and turn the lights off? | _____ hours _____ minutes |
| On a typical night (past month), how many times do you wake up during the middle of the night? | _____ times |
| What wakes you up at night? (circle any that apply) pain, noise, nocturia, child, spontaneous | |
| On a typical night, how long do you spend awake in the middle of the night (total no. of minutes/hours for all awakenings)? | _____ hours _____ minutes |
| How many hours of sleep per night do you usually get? | _____ hours _____ minutes |

### 3. Sleeping Aids

In the past 4 weeks have you used sleeping pills?            Yes        No
   Which drugs? Prescribed, over-the-counter, or both?
   What dosage?
   How many nights/week?
If no, have your ever?
When did you *first* use sleep medication?
When did you *last* use sleep medication?

In the past 4 weeks, have you used alcohol as a sleep aid?   Yes        No
   What kind and how many ounces?
   How many nights/week?
If no, have you ever?

### 4. Sleeping Problem History (onset, course, duration)

How long have you been suffering from insomnia?        _____ years _____ months
Were there any stressful life events related to its onset
   (e.g., death of a loved one, divorce, retirement,
   medical or emotional problems, etc.)?
Gradual or sudden onset?
What has been the course of your insomnia problem
   since its onset (e.g., persistent, episodic, seasonal,
   etc.)?

### 5. Bedroom Environment

| | | |
|---|---|---|
| Are you sleeping with a bed partner? | Yes | No |
| Is your mattress comfortable? | Yes | No |
| Is your bedroom quiet? | Yes | No |
| Do you have a TV, radio, or phone in your bedroom? | Yes | No |
| Is there a desk with paperwork to be done in the bedroom? | Yes | No |
| Do you read in bed before bedtime? | Yes | No |

What is your room temperature at night?

### 6. Eating, Exercise, and Substance Use Habits

How many times per week do you exercise?
Do you sometimes exercise prior to bedtime?            Yes        No
How many caffeinated beverages do you drink per day?
   After dinner?
How many cigarettes per day do you smoke?
How many ounces of alcohol per day do you drink?
Liquid intake in the evening?

7. *Functional Analysis*

What is your prebedtime routine like?

What do you do when you can't fall asleep or return to sleep?

Is your sleep better/worse/same when you go away from home?

Is your sleep better/worse/same on weekends?

What types of factors exacerbate your sleep problem (e.g., stress at work, travel plan, etc.)?

What types of factors improve sleep (e.g., vacation, sex, etc.)?

How concerned are you about sleep/insomnia?

What impact does insomnia have on your life (mood, alertness, performance)?

How do you cope with these daytime sequelae?

Have you received treatment in the past other than sleeping aids?

What prompted you to seek insomnia treatment at this time?

8. *Symptoms of Other Sleep Disorders*

Have you or your spouse ever noticed one of the following, and if so, how often on a typical week would you say you experience these symptoms?

A. *Restless legs*: Crawling or aching feelings in the legs (calves) and inability to keep legs still.

B. *Periodic limb movements*: Leg twitches or jerks during the night; waking up with cramps in legs.

C. *Apnea*: Snoring, pauses in breathing at night, shortness of breath, choking at night; morning headaches, chest pain, dry mouth.

D. *Narcolepsy*: Sleep attacks, sleep paralysis, hypnagogic hallucinations, cataplexy.

E. *Gastro-esophageal reflux*: Sour taste in mouth, heartburn; reflux.

F. *Parasomnias*: Nightmares, night terrors, sleepwalking/talking, bruxism.

G. *Sleep–wake schedule disorder*: Rotating shift or night shift work.

*Diagnostic Impression*:

9. *Medical History/Medication Use*

Last physical exam:                                    Weight:        Height:

Current medical problems:

Current medications:

Hospitalizations/surgery:

10. *History of Psychopathology/Psychiatric Treatment*

(Adapted from the Structured Clinical Interview for DSM-III-R [SCID])

Are you currently receiving psychological or psychiatric treat-      Yes        No
ment for emotional or mental health problems?

Have you or anyone in your family ever been treated for             Yes        No
emotional or mental health problems in the past?

| | | | | | |
|---|---|---|---|---|---|
| Have you or anyone in your family ever been a patient in a psychiatric hospital? | Yes | | No | | |
| Has alcohol or any drug ever caused a problem for you? | Yes | | No | | |
| Have you ever been treated for alcohol/substance abuse problems? | Yes | | No | | |
| Has anything happened lately that has been especially hard for you? | Yes | | No | | |
| What about difficulties at work or with your family? | Yes | | No | | |
| In the last month, has there been a period of time when you were feeling depressed or down most of the day nearly every day? If yes, as long as 2 weeks? | ? | 1 | 2 | 3 | |
| What about being a lot less interested in most things or unable to enjoy the things you used to enjoy? If yes, was it nearly every day? | ? | 1 | 2 | 3 | |
| For the past couple of years, have you been bothered by depressed mood most of the day, more days than not? More than half the time? | ? | 1 | 2 | 3 | |
| Have you ever had a panic attack, when you suddenly felt frightened, anxious or extremely uncomfortable? If yes, 4 attacks within 1 month? | ? | 1 | 2 | 3 | |
| Have you ever been afraid of going out of the house alone, being in crowds, standing in a line, or traveling on buses or trains? | ? | 1 | 2 | 3 | |
| Have you ever been bothered by thoughts that didn't make any sense and kept coming back to you even when you tried not to have them? | ? | 1 | 2 | 3 | |
| In the last 6 months, have you been particularly nervous or anxious? | ? | 1 | 2 | 3 | |
| Do you worry a lot about terrible things that might happen? | ? | 1 | 2 | 3 | |
| During the last 6 months, would you say that you have been worrying most of the time (more days than not)? | ? | 1 | 2 | 3 | |
| If psychopathology is present, evaluate its onset and temporal course in relation to the sleep disturbance. | | | | | |
| Does insomnia occur exclusively during the course of anxiety/depression episodes? | Yes | | No | | |

*Diagnostic Impression:*

? = Inadequate information   1 = Absent or false   2 = Subthreshold   3 = Present

## APPENDIX B. Sleep Impairment Index

1. Please rate the current severity of your insomnia problem(s):

| | None | Mild | Moderate | Severe | Very |
|---|---|---|---|---|---|
| Difficulty falling asleep: | 1 | 2 | 3 | 4 | 5 |
| Difficulty staying asleep: | 1 | 2 | 3 | 4 | 5 |
| Problem waking up too early: | 1 | 2 | 3 | 4 | 5 |

2. How satisfied/dissatisfied are you with your current sleep pattern?

| Very satisfied | | Moderately satisfied | | Very dissatisfied |
|---|---|---|---|---|
| 1 | 2 | 3 | 4 | 5 |

3. To what extent do you consider your sleep problem to INTERFERE with your daily functioning (e.g., daytime fatigue, ability to function at work/daily chores, concentration, memory, mood, etc.)?

| Not at all | A little | Somewhat | Much | Very much |
|---|---|---|---|---|
| 1 | 2 | 3 | 4 | 5 |

4. How NOTICEABLE to others do you think your sleeping problem is in terms of impairing the quality of your life?

| Not at all | A little | Somewhat | Much | Very much |
|---|---|---|---|---|
| 1 | 2 | 3 | 4 | 5 |

5. How CONCERNED are you about your current sleep problem?

| Not at all | A little | Somewhat | Much | Very much |
|---|---|---|---|---|
| 1 | 2 | 3 | 4 | 5 |

6. To what extent do you believe the following factors are contributing to your sleep problem?

| | None | | Some | | Much |
|---|---|---|---|---|---|
| Cognitive disturbances (racing thoughts at night): | 1 | 2 | 3 | 4 | 5 |
| Somatic disturbances (muscular tension; pain): | 1 | 2 | 3 | 4 | 5 |
| Bad sleeping habits: | 1 | 2 | 3 | 4 | 5 |
| Natural aging processes: | 1 | 2 | 3 | 4 | 5 |

7. After a poor night's sleep, which of the following problems do you experience on the next day? Circle all those that apply.

   a. Daytime fatigue: tired, exhausted, washed out, sleepy.
   b. Difficulty functioning: performance impairment at work/daily chores, difficulty concentrating, memory problems.
   c. Mood problems: irritable, tense, nervous, groggy, depressed, anxious, grouchy, hostile, angry, confused.
   d. Physical symptoms: muscle aches/pain, light-headed, headache, nausea, heartburn, muscle tension.
   e. None

## APPENDIX C. Beliefs and Attitudes about Sleep Scale

Several statements reflecting people's beliefs and attitudes about sleep are listed below. Please indicate to what extent you personally agree or disagree with each statement. There is no right or wrong answer. For each statement, place a mark (/) along the line wherever your *personal* rating falls. Try to use the whole scale, rather than placing your marks at one end of the line.

1. I need 8 hours of sleep to feel refreshed and function well during the day.

   Strongly _____ Strongly
   disagree                                            agree

2. When I don't get a proper amount of sleep on a given night, I need to catch up on the next day by napping or on the next night by sleeping longer.

   Strongly _____ Strongly
   disagree                                            agree

3. Because I am getting older, I need less sleep.

   Strongly _____ Strongly
   disagree                                            agree

4. I am worried that if I go for one or two nights without sleep, I may have a nervous breakdown.

   Strongly _____ Strongly
   disagree                                            agree

5. I am concerned that chronic insomnia may have serious consequences for my physical health.

   Strongly _____ Strongly
   disagree                                            agree

6. By spending more time in bed, I usually get more sleep and feel better the next day.

   Strongly _____ Strongly
   disagree                                            agree

7. When I have trouble getting to sleep, I should stay in bed and try harder.

   Strongly _____ Strongly
   disagree                                            agree

8. I am worried that I may lose control over my abilities to sleep.

Strongly _____ Strongly
disagree                                                    agree

9. Because I am getting older, I should go to bed earlier in the evening.

Strongly _____ Strongly
disagree                                                    agree

10. After a poor night's sleep, I know that it will interfere with my daily activities on the next day.

Strongly _____ Strongly
disagree                                                    agree

11. In order to be alert and function well during the day, I am better off taking a sleeping pill rather than having a poor night's sleep.

Strongly _____ Strongly
disagree                                                    agree

12. When I feel irritable, depressed, or anxious during the day, it is mostly because I did not sleep well the night before.

Strongly _____ Strongly
disagree                                                    agree

13. Because my bed partner falls asleep as soon as his or her head hits the pillow and stays asleep through the night, I should be able to do so too.

Strongly _____ Strongly
disagree                                                    agree

14. I feel that insomnia is basically the result of aging, and there isn't much that can be done about this problem.

Strongly _____ Strongly
disagree                                                    agree

15. I am sometimes afraid of dying in my sleep.

Strongly _____ Strongly
disagree                                                    agree

16. When I have a good night's sleep, I know that I will have to pay for it on the following night.

Strongly _____ Strongly
disagree                                                    agree

17. When I sleep poorly on one night, I know it will disturb my sleep schedule for the whole week.

Strongly _____ Strongly
disagree                                                                              agree

18. Without an adequate night's sleep, I can hardly function the next day.

Strongly _____ Strongly
disagree                                                                              agree

19. I can't ever predict whether I'll have a good or poor night's sleep.

Strongly _____ Strongly
disagree                                                                              agree

20. I have little ability to manage the negative consequences of disturbed sleep.

Strongly _____ Strongly
disagree                                                                              agree

21. When I feel tired, have no energy, or just seem not to function well during the day, it is generally because I did not sleep well the night before.

Strongly _____ Strongly
disagree                                                                              agree

22. I get overwhelmed by my thoughts at night and often feel I have no control over my racing mind.

Strongly _____ Strongly
disagree                                                                              agree

23. I feel I can still lead a satisfactory life despite sleep difficulties.

Strongly _____ Strongly
disagree                                                                              agree

24. I believe insomnia is essentially the result of a chemical imbalance.

Strongly _____ Strongly
disagree                                                                              agree

25. I feel insomnia is ruining my ability to enjoy life and prevents me from doing what I want.

Strongly _____ Strongly
disagree                                                                              agree

26. I avoid or cancel obligations (social, family, occupational) after a poor night's sleep.

Strongly _____ Strongly
disagree                                                                      agree

27. A "nightcap" before bedtime is a good solution to sleep problems.

Strongly _____ Strongly
disagree                                                                      agree

28. Medication is probably the only solution to sleeplessness.

Strongly _____ Strongly
disagree                                                                      agree

29. My sleep is getting worse all the time, and I don't believe anyone can help.

Strongly _____ Strongly
disagree                                                                      agree

30. It usually shows in my physical appearance when I haven't slept well.

Strongly _____ Strongly
disagree                                                                      agree

## APPENDIX D. Insomnia Treatment Acceptability Scale

Two treatment methods commonly used for insomnia problems are described below. Please read the description of each method and answer each question as it would apply to your insomnia problem. For each question, place a mark (/) somewhere along the continuous line wherever your *personal* rating falls. Please consider the line to represent your own personal range. Try to use the whole scale, rather than simply putting your marks at one end or the other.

Example: I usually have trouble falling asleep.

Not at all _____/_____ Very much

*Treatment 1: Behavioral Treatment*

This is a nondrug treatment method aimed at teaching patients self-management skills to overcome insomnia. The behavioral component provides specific guidelines for changing poor sleep habits and for regulating sleep schedules. Patients are also guided to examine and modify their beliefs and attitudes about sleep that may perpetuate their insomnia. Education about sleep hygiene factors (e.g., diet, exercise, and substance use) is also provided.

Please complete all your ratings for this treatment method before proceeding to read the description of the second treatment method.

1. How acceptable would you consider this treatment for your insomnia?

Not at all _____ Very
acceptable                                                acceptable

2. How acceptable would you consider this treatment for other people with insomnia?

Not at all _____ Very
acceptable                                                acceptable

3. How willing would you be to adhere to this treatment regimen if recommended for your insomnia?

Not at all _____ Very
willing                                                   willing

4. How suitable do you think this treatment would be for treating:
(A) Difficulty falling asleep at bedtime?

Not at all _____ Very
suitable                                                  suitable

(B) Difficulty staying asleep during the night?

Not at all _____ Very
suitable                                                                   suitable

5. How effective do you believe this treatment would be in the short term?

Not at all _____ Very
effective                                                                 effective

6. How effective do you believe this treatment would be for producing a permanent cure?

Not at all _____ Very
effective                                                                 effective

7. In addition to improving sleep, how effective would this treatment be for improving other aspects of your daytime functioning (e.g., alertness, performance, mood)?

Not at all _____ Very
effective                                                                 effective

8. To what extent would this treatment produce side effects?
Very strong _____ No
side effects                                                              side effects


*Treatment 2: Pharmacological Treatment*

This drug treatment consists of taking a prescribed sleeping pill at bedtime. The prescribed hypnotic medication is specifically designed to produce a state of relaxation by reducing physiological (muscular) and cognitive (mental) arousal at bedtime. This medication also increases the threshold for awakening at night and makes patients less sensitive to factors that usually wake them up at night. The specific type of medication and dosage would be based on the nature and severity of the insomnia problem.

1. How acceptable would you consider this treatment for your insomnia?

Not at all _____ Very
acceptable                                                                acceptable

2. How acceptable would you consider this treatment for other people with insomnia?

Not at all _____ Very
acceptable                                                                acceptable

3. How willing would you be to adhere to this treatment regimen if recommended for your insomnia?

Not at all   _____   Very
willing                                                        willing

4. How suitable do you think this treatment would be for treating:
   (A) Difficulty falling asleep at bedtime?

Not at all   _____   Very
suitable                                                   suitable

   (B) Difficulty staying asleep during the night?

Not at all   _____   Very
suitable                                                   suitable

5. How effective do you believe this treatment would be in the short term?

Not at all   _____   Very
effective                                                 effective

6. How effective do you believe this treatment would be for producing a permanent cure?

Not at all   _____   Very
effective                                                 effective

7. In addition to improving sleep, how effective would this treatment be for improving other aspects of your daytime functioning (e.g., alertness, performance, mood)?

Not at all   _____   Very
effective                                                 effective

8. To what extent would this treatment produce side effects?

Very strong   _____   No
side effects                                               side effects

## APPENDIX E. Personal Contract

This is a personal contract between you, the patient, and your therapist. This contract explains what is expected from both parties during the treatment program. It is intended to promote systematic and consistent adherence to newly learned self-management skills for overcoming insomnia.

I understand that I will be offered a comprehensive treatment program for insomnia, which will include three main components and a fourth optional one.

  a. *Behavioral*: This component is aimed at providing me with specific guidelines for changing maladaptive sleep habits that perpetuate my difficulties initiating/maintaining sleep.
  b. *Cognitive*: This component is aimed at helping me reframe some of my beliefs and attitudes about sleeplessness, which may feed into my insomnia problem.
  c. *Educational*: This component is aimed at providing me with information on basic facts about sleep and changes in sleep patterns over the course of the lifespan. It is intended to teach me sleep hygiene principles about the effects of diet, exercise, and substance use (e.g., caffeine, alcohol) on sleep.
  d. *Medication*: This component (if applicable) will provide me with a schedule to follow to gradually discontinue use of sleep medication.

This is a time-limited treatment program, which will provide me with information, support, and training for developing self-management skills aimed at overcoming/coping with insomnia.

In return, I personally agree to:

  a. Attend between 8 and 10 weekly therapy sessions.
  b. Complete my diary on a daily basis for the duration of treatment.
  c. Carefully follow the treatment recommendations and homework assignments.
  d. Use sleep medication only as recommended.
  e. Complete several questionnaires before and after treatment.

Patient: _____     Date: _____

Therapist: _____     Date: _____

## APPENDIX F. Sleep Diary

### INSTRUCTIONS

In order to better understand your sleep problem and monitor your progress during treatment, we would like you to collect some important information on your sleep pattern. After you get up in the morning, please answer all 10 questions on the sleep diary. It is important that you complete this diary *every morning*. For example, when you get up on a Wednesday morning, complete the column under Tuesday; on a Thursday morning, complete the column under Wednesday; and so forth. It is difficult to estimate how long you take to fall asleep or how long you are awake at night. Please remember, however, that we only want your best *estimates*. If there should be some unusual event on a given night (e.g., illness, emergency, phone call), make a note of it. Below are some guidelines to help you answer each question. An example is also provided on the diary.

1. *Napping:* This should include all naps even though they were not intentional. For instance, if you dozed off in front of the TV for 10 minutes, please write this down. Make sure to specify A.M. or P.M.
2. *Sleep Aid:* You should include both prescribed and over-the-counter medications, as well as alcohol used specifically as a sleep aid.
3. *Bedtime:* This is the time you go to bed and actually turn the lights off. If you go to bed at 10:45 but turn the lights off only at 11:15, you should write both times in that space.
4. *Sleep-Onset Latency:* Provide your best *estimate* of how long it took you to fall asleep after you turned the lights off and intended to go to sleep.
5. *Number of Awakenings:* This is the number of times you remember waking up during the night.
6. *Duration of Awakenings:* Please estimate to the best of your knowledge how many minutes you spent awake for each awakening. If this proved impossible, then estimate the number of minutes you spent awake for all awakenings combined. This should not include your very last awakening in the morning, as this will be logged in number 7.
7. *Morning Awakening:* This is the very last time you woke up in the morning. If you woke up at 4:00 and never went back to sleep, this is the time to write. However, if you woke up at 4:00 but went back to sleep for a brief period of time (for example, from 6:00 to 6:20), then your last awakening would be 6:20.
8. *Out-of-Bed Time:* This is the time you actually got out of bed for the day.
9. *Feeling upon Arising:* Please use the following 5-point scale:
   1 = Exhausted; 2 = Tired; 3 = Average; 4 = Rather refreshed; 5 = Very refreshed.
10. *Sleep Quality:* Please use the following 5-point scale:
   1 = Very restless; 2 = Restless; 3 = Average quality; 4 = Sound; 5 = Very sound.

SLEEP DIARY

| | Example | Mon | Tue | Wed | Thu | Fri | Sat | Sun |
|---|---|---|---|---|---|---|---|---|
| 1. Yesterday, I napped from —— to —— (note the times of all naps). | 1:50 to 2:30 p.m. | | | | | | | |
| 2. Yesterday, I took —— mg of medication and/or —— oz of —— alcohol as a sleep aid. | Ambien 5 mg | | | | | | | |
| 3. Last night, I went to bed and turned the lights off at —— o'clock. | 11:15 | | | | | | | |
| 4. After turning the lights out, I fell asleep in —— minutes. | 40 min | | | | | | | |
| 5. My sleep was interrupted —— times (specify number of nighttime awakenings). | 3 | | | | | | | |
| 6. My sleep was interrupted for —— minutes (specify duration of each awakening). | 10 5 45 | | | | | | | |
| 7. This morning, I woke up at —— o'clock (note time of last awakening). | 6:15 | | | | | | | |
| 8. This morning, I got out of bed at —— o'clock (specify the time). | 6:40 | | | | | | | |
| 9. When I got up this morning I felt ——. (1 = exhausted, 5 = refreshed) | 2 | | | | | | | |
| 10. Overall, my sleep last night was ——. (1 = very restless, 5 = very sound) | 3 | | | | | | | |

## APPENDIX G. Summary of Sleep Diary Data

| Date | Week | SOL | WASO | EMA | TWT | TST | TIB | SE | FNA | Comments |
|------|------|-----|------|-----|-----|-----|-----|----|-----|----------|
| | 1 | | | | | | | | | |
| | 2 | | | | | | | | | |
| X̄ Pretreatment: | | | | | | | | | | |
| | 3 | | | | | | | | | |
| | 4 | | | | | | | | | |
| | 5 | | | | | | | | | |
| | 6 | | | | | | | | | |
| X̄ Midtreatment: | | | | | | | | | | |
| | 7 | | | | | | | | | |
| | 8 | | | | | | | | | |
| | 9 | | | | | | | | | |
| | 10 | | | | | | | | | |
| X̄ Posttreatment: | | | | | | | | | | |
| X̄ Follow-up: | | | | | | | | | | |

*Note.* SOL, sleep-onset latency; WASO, wake after sleep onset; EMA, early morning awakening; TWT, total wake time (SOL + WASO + EMA); TST, total sleep time; TIB, time in bed; SE, sleep efficiency (TST/TIB × 100); FNA, frequency of night awakenings.

# References

Aber, R., & Webb, W. B. (1986). Effects of a limited nap on night sleep in older subjects. *Psychology and Aging*, 4, 300–302.

Adam, K. (1980). Dietary habit and sleep after bedtime food drinks. *Sleep*, 3, 47–58.

Adam, K., & Oswald, I. (1989). Can a rapidly-eliminated hypnotic cause daytime anxiety? *Pharmacopsychiatry*, 22, 115–119.

Allen, R. P. (1991). Early morning awakening insomnia: Bright-light treatment. In P. Hauri (Ed.), *Case studies in insomnia* (pp. 207–220). New York: Plenum Press.

Allen, R. P., Mendels, J., Nevins, D. B., Chernik, D. A., & Hoddes, E. (1987). Efficacy without tolerance or rebound insomnia for midazolam and temazepam after use for one to three months. *Journal of Clinical Pharmacology*, 27, 768–775.

Alperson, J., & Biglan, A. (1979). Self-administered treatment of sleep onset insomnia and the importance of age. *Behavior Therapy*, 10, 347–356.

American Psychiatric Association (APA). (in press). *Diagnostic and statistical manual of mental disorders* (4th ed). Washington, DC: Author.

American Sleep Disorders Association (ASDA). (1990). *International classification of sleep disorders: Diagnostic and coding manual*. Rochester, MN: Author.

Ancoli-Israel, S., Kripke, D. F., Mason, W., & Kaplan, O. J. (1985). Sleep apnea and periodic movements in sleep in an aging population. *Journal of Gerontology*, 40, 419–425.

Ancoli-Israel, S., Kripke, D. F., Mason, W., & Messin, S. (1981). Sleep apnea and nocturnal myoclonus in a senior population. *Sleep*, 4, 349–358.

Ascher, L. M., & Efran, J. S. (1978). Use of paradoxical intention in a behavioral program for sleep onset insomnia. *Journal of Consulting and Clinical Psychology*, 46, 547–550.

Ascher, L. M., & Turner, R. M. (1979). Paradoxical intention and insomnia: An experimental investigation. *Behaviour Research and Therapy*, 17, 408–411.

Association of Sleep Disorders Centers. (1979). Diagnostic classification of sleep and arousal disorders. *Sleep*, 2, 1–137.

Atkinson, J. H., Ancoli-Israel, S., Slater, M. A., Garfin, S. R., & Gillin, J. C. (1988). Subjective sleep disturbance in chronic back pain. *Clinical Journal of Pain*, 4, 225–232.

Ballinger, C. B. (1976). Subjective sleep disturbance at the menopause. *Journal of Psychosomatic Research*, 20, 509–513.

Balter, M. B., & Uhlenhuth, E. H. (1991). The beneficial and adverse effects of hypnotics. *Journal of Clinical Psychiatry*, 52(Suppl.), 16–23.

Barratt, E. S., Beaver, W., & White, R. (1974). The effects of marijuana on human sleep patterns. *Biological Psychology*, 8, 47–54.

Beck, A. T., Emery, G., & Greenberg, R. L. (1985). *Anxiety disorders and phobias: A cognitive perspective.* New York: Basic Books.

Beck, A. T., Epstein, N., Brown, G., & Steer, R. (1988). An inventory for measuring clinical anxiety: Psychometric properties. *Journal of Consulting and Clinical Psychology, 56,* 893–897.

Beck, A. T., Rush, A. J., Shaw, B. F., & Emery, G. (1979). *Cognitive therapy of depression.* New York: Guilford Press.

Beck, A. T., Ward, C. H., Mendelson, M., Mock, J., & Erbaugh, J. (1961). An inventory for measuring depression. *Archives of General Psychiatry, 4,* 561–571.

Bédard, M. A., Montplaisir, J., Richer, F., Rouleau, I., & Malo, J. (1991). Obstructive sleep apnea syndrome: Pathogenesis of neuropsychological deficits. *Journal of Clinical and Experimental Neuropsychology, 13,* 950–964.

Berlin, R. M. (1984). Management of insomnia in hospitalized patients. *Annals of Internal Medicine, 100,* 398–404.

Berlin, R. M., Litovitz, G. L., Diaz, M. A., & Ahmed, S. W. (1984). Sleep disorders on a psychiatric consultation service. *American Journal of Psychiatry, 141,* 582–584.

Berntzen, D., & Gotestam, K. G. (1987). Effects of on-demand versus fixed-interval schedules in the treatment of chronic pain with analgesic compounds. *Journal of Consulting and Clinical Psychology, 55,* 213–217.

Betts, T. A., & Alford, C. (1983). Beta-blocking drugs and sleep. *Drugs, 25,* 268–272.

Birrell, P. C. (1983). Behavioral, subjective, and electroencephalographic indices of sleep onset latency and sleep duration. *Journal of Behavioral Assessment, 5,* 179–190.

Bixler, E. O., Kales, A., & Soldatos, C. R. (1979). Sleep disorders encountered in medical practice: A national survey of physicians. *Behavioral Medicine, 6,* 1–6.

Bixler, E. O., Kales, A., Soldatos, C. R., Kales, J. D., & Healy, B. (1979). Prevalence of sleep disorders in the Los Angeles metropolitan area. *American Journal of Psychiatry, 136,* 1257–1262.

Bixler, E. O., Kales, A., Soldatos, C. R., Scharf, M. B., & Kales, J. D. (1978). Effectiveness of temazepam with short-, intermediate-, and long-term use: Sleep laboratory evaluation. *Journal of Clinical Pharmacology, 18,* 110–118.

Bliwise, D. L. (1989). Neuropsychological function and sleep. *Clinics in Geriatric Medicine, 5,* 381–394.

Bliwise, D. L., King, A. C., Harris, R., & Haskell, W. (1992). Prevalence of self-reported poor sleep in a healthy population aged 50–65. *Social Sciences and Medicine, 34,* 49–55.

Bliwise, D. L., Seidel, W. F., Greenblatt, D. J., & Dement, W. C. (1984). Nighttime and daytime efficacy of flurazepam and oxazepam in chronic insomnia. *American Journal of Psychiatry, 141,* 191–195.

Bonnet, M. H. (1983). Memory for events occurring during arousal from sleep. *Psychophysiology, 20,* 81–87.

Bootzin, R. R. (1972). Stimulus control treatment for insomnia. *Proceedings of the American Psychological Association, 7,* 395–396.

Bootzin, R. R. (1985). Insomnia. In M. Hersen & C. Last (Eds.), *Behavior therapy casebook* (pp. 132–143). New York: Springer.

Bootzin, R. R., & Engle-Friedman, M. E. (1981). The assessment of insomnia. *Behavioral Assessment, 3,* 107–126.

Bootzin, R. R., Engle-Friedman, M. E., & Hazelwood, L. (1983). Insomnia. In P. M. Lewinsohn & L. Teri (Eds.), *Clinical geropsychology: New directions in assessment and treatment* (pp. 81–115). Elmsford, NY: Pergamon Press.

Bootzin, R. R., Epstein, D., & Wood, J. M. (1991). Stimulus control instructions. In P. Hauri (Ed.), *Case studies in insomnia* (pp. 19–28). New York: Plenum Press.

Bootzin, R. R., Herman, C. P., & Nicassio, P. M. (1976). The power of suggestion: Another examination of misattribution and insomnia. *Journal of Personality and Social Psychology*, *34*, 673–679.

Bootzin, R. R., & Nicassio, P. M. (1978). Behavioral treatments of insomnia. In M. Hersen, R. E. Eisler, & P. M. Miller (Eds.), *Progress in behavior modification* (Vol. 6, pp. 1–45). New York: Academic Press.

Borkovec, T. D. (1979). Pseudo (experiential)-insomnia and idiopathic (objective) insomnia: Theoretical and therapeutic issues. *Advances in Behaviour Research and Therapy*, *2*, 27–55.

Borkovec, T. D. (1982). Insomnia. *Journal of Consulting and Clinical Psychology*, *50*, 880–895.

Borkovec, T. D., Grayson, T. T., O'Brien, G. T., & Weerts, T. C. (1979). Relaxation treatment of pseudo insomnia and idiopathic insomnia: An electroencephalographic evaluation. *Journal of Applied Behavior Analysis*, *12*, 37–54.

Borkovec, T. D., Lane, T. W., & Van Oot, P. H. (1981). Phenomenology of sleep among insomniacs and good sleepers: Wakefulness experience when cortically asleep. *Journal of Abnormal Psychology*, *90*, 607–609.

Borkovec, T. D., & Weerts, T. C. (1976). Effects of progressive relaxation on sleep disturbances: An electroencephalographic evaluation. *Psychosomatic Medicine*, *38*, 173–180.

Browman, C. P. (1980). Sleep following sustained exercise. *Psychophysiology*, *6*, 577–580.

Buela-Casal, G., Sierra, J. C., & Caballo, V. E. (1992). Personality differences between short and long sleepers. *Personality and Individual Differences*, *13*, 115–117.

Bunnell, D. E., Agnew, J. A., Horvath, S. M., Jopson, L., & Wills, M. (1988). Passive body heating and sleep: Influence of proximity to sleep. *Sleep*, *11*, 210–219.

Bunnell, D. E., Bevier, W., & Horvath, S. M. (1983). Effects of exhaustive exercise on the sleep of men and women. *Psychophysiology*, *1*, 50–58.

Burnett, K. F., Taylor, C. B., Thoresen, C. E., Rosekind, M. R., Miles, L. E., & DeBusk, R. F. (1985). Toward computerized scoring of sleep using ambulatory recordings of heart rate and physical activity. *Behavioral Assessment*, *7*, 261–271.

Buysse, D. J., Reynolds, C. F., Monk, T. H., Berman, S. R., & Kupfer, D. J. (1989). The Pittsburgh Sleep Quality Index: A new instrument for psychiatric practice and research. *Psychiatry Research*, *28*, 193–213.

Cannici, J., Malcolm, R., & Peek, L. (1983). Treatment of insomnia in cancer patients using muscle relaxation training. *Journal of Behavior Therapy and Experimental Psychiatry*, *14*, 251–256.

Carney, R. M., Freedland, K. E., & Jaffe, A. S. (1990). Insomnia and depression prior to myocardial infarction. *Psychosomatic Medicine*, *52*, 603–609.

Carr-Kaffashan, L., & Woolfolk, R. L. (1979). Active and placebo effects in the treatment of moderate and severe insomnia. *Journal of Consulting and Clinical Psychology*, *47*, 1072–1080.

Carrera, R. N., & Elenewski, J. J. (1980). Implosive therapy as a treatment for insomnia. *Journal of Clinical Psychology*, *36*, 729–734.

Carskadon, M. A., & Dement, W. C. (1989). Normal sleep and its variations. In M. H. Kryger, T. Roth, & W. C. Dement (Eds.), *Principles and practice of sleep medicine* (pp. 3–13). Philadelphia: Saunders.

Carskadon, M. A., Dement, W. C., Mitler, M. M., Guilleminault, C., Zarcone, V., & Spiegel, R. (1976). Self-report versus sleep laboratory findings in 122 drug-free subjects with complaints of insomnia. *American Journal of Psychiatry*, *133*, 1382–1388.

Carskadon, M. A., & Rechtschaffen, A. (1989). Monitoring and staging human sleep. In M. H. Kryger, T. Roth, & W. C. Dement (Eds.), *Principles and practice of sleep medicine* (pp. 665–683). Philadelphia: Saunders.

Carskadon, M. A., Seidel, W. F., Greenblatt, D. J., & Dement, W. C. (1982). Daytime carry-over of triazolam and flurazepam in elderly insomniacs. *Sleep*, *5*, 361–371.

Carter, W. R., Johnson, M. C., & Borkovec, T. D. (1986). Worry: An electrocortical analysis. *Behaviour Research and Therapy*, 8, 193–204.

Cashman, M. A., & McCann, B. S. (1988). Behavioral approaches to sleep/wake disorders in children and adolescents. In M. Hersen, R. E. Eisler, & P. M. Miller (Eds.), *Progress in behavior modification* (Vol. 22, pp. 215–283). New York: Academic Press.

Chambers, M. J. (1992). Therapeutic issues in the behavioral treatment of insomnia. *Professional Psychology: Research and Practice*, 23, 131–138.

Church, M. W., & Johnson, L. C. (1979). Mood and performance of poor sleepers during repeated use of flurazepam. *Psychopharmacology*, 61, 309–316.

Coates, T. J., Killen, J. D., George, J., Marchini, E., Silverman, S., & Thoresen, C. E. (1982). Estimating sleep parameters: A multitrait–multimethod analysis. *Journal of Consulting and Clinical Psychology*, 50, 345–352.

Coates, T. J., Killen, J. D., Silverman, S., George, J., Marchini, E., Hamilton, S., & Thoresen, C. E. (1983). Cognitive activity, sleep disturbance, and stage specific differences between recorded and reported sleep. *Psychophysiology*, 20, 243–250.

Coates, T. J., & Thoresen, C. E. (1981). Sleep disturbance in children and adolescents. In E. G. Mash & L. G. Terdal (Eds.), *Behavioral assessment of childhood disorders* (pp. 639–678). New York: Guilford Press.

Coleman, R. M., Roffwarg, H. P., Kennedy, S. J., Guilleminault, C., Cinque, J., Cohn, M. A., Karacan, I., Kupfer, D. J., Lemmi, H., Miles, L. E., Orr, W. C., Phillips, E. R., Roth, T., Sassin, J. F., Schmidt, H. S., Weitzman, E. D., & Dement, W. C. (1982). Sleep–wake disorders based on a polysomnographic diagnosis: A national cooperative study. *Journal of the American Medical Association*, 247, 997–1003.

Coren, S. (1988). Prediction of insomnia from arousability predisposition scores: Scale development and cross-validation. *Behaviour Research and Therapy*, 26, 415–420.

Coren, S., & Searleman, A. (1985). Birth stress and self-reported sleep difficulty. *Sleep*, 8, 222–226.

Coren, S., & Ward, L. M. (1989). *Sensation and perception* (3rd ed.). San Diego: Harcourt Brace Jovanovich.

Coursey, R. D., Frankel, B. L., Gaardner, K. B., & Moot, D. E. (1980). A comparison of relaxation techniques with electrosleep therapy for chronic sleep-onset insomnia: A sleep EEG study. *Biofeedback and Self-Regulation*, 5, 57–73.

Coyle, K., & Watts, F. N. (1991). The factorial structure of sleep dissatisfaction. *Behaviour Research and Therapy*, 29, 513–520.

Crisp, A. H., Stonehill, E., Fenton, G. W., & Fenwick, P. B. (1973). Sleep patterns in obese patients during weight reduction. *Psychotherapy and Psychosomatics*, 22, 159–165.

Curatolo, P. W., & Robertson, D. (1983). The health consequences of caffeine. *Annals of Internal Medicine*, 5, 641–653.

Czeisler, C. A., Johnson, M., Duffy, J., Brown, E., Ronda, J., & Kronauer, R. (1990). Exposure to bright light and darkness to treat physiologic maladaptation to night work. *New England Journal of Medicine*, 322, 1253–1259.

Czeisler, C. A., Richardson, G. S., Coleman, R. M., Zimmerman, J. C., Moore-Ede, M. C., Dement, W. C., & Weitzman, E. D. (1981). Chronotherapy: Resetting the circadian clocks of patients with delayed sleep phase insomnia. *Sleep*, 4, 1–21.

Czeisler, C. A., Weitzman, E. D., Moore-Ede, M. C., Zimmerman, J. C., & Knauer, R. (1980). Human sleep: Its duration and organization depend on its circadian phase. *Science*, 210, 1264–1267.

Davidson, G. C., Tsujimoto, R. N., & Glaros, A. G. (1973). Attribution and the maintenance of behavior change in falling asleep. *Journal of Abnormal Psychology*, 82, 124–133.

Davidson, R. J. (1978). Specificity and patterning in biobehavioral systems: Implications for behavioral change. *American Psychologist*, 33, 430–436.

Davies, R., Lacks, P., Storandt, M., & Bertelson, A. D. (1986). Counter-control treatment of sleep-maintenance insomnia in relation to age. *Psychology and Aging, 1,* 233–238.

Dement, W. C. Foreword. (1991a). In P. Hauri (Ed.), *Case studies in insomnia* (p. vii). New York: Plenum Press.

Dement, W. C. (1991b). Objective measurements of daytime sleepiness and performance comparing quazepam with flurazepam in two adult populations using the Multiple Sleep Latency Test. *Journal of Clinical Psychiatry, 52*(Suppl.), 31–37.

Dement, W. C., Miles, L. E., & Carskadon, M. A. (1982). "White paper" on sleep and aging. *Journal of the American Geriatrics Society, 30,* 25–50.

Dement, W. C., Seidel, W. F., & Carskadon, M. A. (1982). Daytime alertness, insomnia and benzodiazepines. *Sleep, 5,* S28–S45.

Derogatis, L. R., & Melisaratos, N. (1983). The Brief Symptom Inventory: An introductory report. *Psychological Medicine, 13,* 595–605.

Downey, R., & Bonnet, M. H. (1992). Training subjective insomniacs to accurately perceive sleep onset. *Sleep, 15,* 58–63.

Edelstein, B., Keaton-Brasted, C., & Burg, M. (1984). Effects of caffeine withdrawal on nocturnal enuresis, insomnia, and behavior restraints. *Journal of Consulting and Clinical Psychology, 52,* 857–862.

Edinger, J. D., Hoelscher, T. J., Marsh, G. R., Lipper, S., & Ionescu-Pioggia, M. (1992). A cognitive-behavioral therapy for sleep-maintenance insomnia in older adults. *Psychology and Aging, 7,* 282–289.

Edinger, J. D., Hoelscher, T. J., Webb, M. D., Marsh, G. R., Radtke, R. A., & Erwin, C. W. (1989). Polysomnographic assessment of DIMS: Empirical evaluation of its diagnostic value. *Sleep, 12,* 315–322.

Edinger, J. D., Lipper, S., & Wheeler, B. (1989). Hospital ward policy and patients' sleep patterns: A multiple baseline study. *Rehabilitation Psychology, 34,* 43–50.

Edinger, J. D., & Stout, A. L. (1985). Efficacy of an outpatient treatment program for insomnia: A preliminary report. *Professional Psychology: Research and Practice, 16,* 905–909.

Edinger, J. D., Stout, A. L., & Hoelscher, T. J. (1988). Cluster analysis of insomniacs' MMPI profiles: Relation of subtypes to sleep history and treatment outcome. *Psychosomatic Medicine, 50,* 77–87.

Engle-Friedman, M., Bootzin, R. R., Hazlewood, L., & Tsao, C. (1992). An evaluation of behavioral treatments for insomnia in the older adult. *Journal of Clinical Psychology, 48,* 77–90.

Espie, C. A. (1991). *The psychological treatment of insomnia.* Chichester, England: Wiley.

Espie, C. A., Brooks, D. N., & Lindsay, W. R. (1989). An evaluation of tailored psychological treatment of insomnia. *Journal of Behavior Therapy and Experimental Psychiatry, 20,* 143–153.

Espie, C. A., & Lindsay, W. R. (1985). Paradoxical intention in the treatment of chronic insomnia: Six case studies illustrating variability in therapeutic response. *Behaviour Research and Therapy, 23,* 703–709.

Espie, C. A., Lindsay, W. R., & Brooks, D. N. (1988). Substituting behavioural treatment for drugs in the treatment of insomnia: An exploratory study. *Journal of Behavior Therapy and Experimental Psychiatry, 19,* 51–56.

Espie, C. A., Lindsay, W. R., Brooks, D. N., Hood, E. M., & Turvey, T. (1989). A controlled comparative investigation of psychological treatments for chronic sleep-onset insomnia. *Behaviour Research and Therapy, 27,* 79–88.

Espie, C. A., Lindsay, W. R., & Espie, L. C. (1989). Use of the Sleep Assessment Device (Kelley and Lichstein, 1980) to validate insomniacs' self-report of sleep pattern. *Journal of Psychopathology and Behavioral Assessment, 11,* 71–79.

Espie, C. A., Monk, E., Hood, E. M., & Lindsay, W. R. (1988). Establishing clinical criteria for the treatment of chronic insomnia: A comparison of insomniac and control populations. *Health Bulletin, 46,* 316–326.

Erman, M. K. (1987). Insomnia. *Psychiatric Clinics of North America, 10,* 525–539.

Evans, L. K. (1987). Sundown syndrome in institutionalized elderly. *Journal of the American Geriatrics Society, 35,* 101–108.

Ferber, R. (1985). *Solve your child's sleep problems.* New York: Simon & Schuster.

Fichten, C. S., & Libman, E. (1991). A new look at the complaint of insomnia and its treatment in older adults. *Santé Mentale au Québec, 16,* 99–116.

Fleming, J. A., McClure, D. J., Mayes, C., Phillips, R., & Bourgouin, J. (1990). A comparison of the efficacy, safety and withdrawal effects of zopiclone and triazolam in the treatment of insomnia. *International Clinical Psychopharmacology, 5*(Suppl.), 29–37.

Follick, M. J., Smith, T. W., & Ahern, D. K. (1985). The Sickness Impact Profile: A global measure of disability in chronic low back pain. *Pain, 21,* 67–76.

Fontaine, R., Beaudry, P., Le Morvan, P., Beauclair, L., & Chouinard, G. (1990). Zopiclone and triazolam in insomnia associated with generalized anxiety disorder: A placebo-controlled evaluation of efficacy and daytime anxiety. *International Clinical Psychopharmacology, 5*(Suppl.), 173–183.

Ford, D. E., & Kamerow, D. B. (1989). Epidemiologic study of sleep disturbances and psychiatric disorders: An opportunity for prevention? *Journal of the American Medical Association, 262,* 1479–1484.

Fraisse, P. (1984). Perception and estimation of time. *Annual Review of Psychology, 35,* 1–36.

Frankel, B. L., Coursey, R., Buchbinder, R., & Snyder, F. (1976). Recorded and reported sleep in primary chronic insomnia. *Archives of General Psychiatry, 33,* 615–623.

Franklin, J. (1981). The measurement of sleep onset latency in insomnia. *Behaviour Research and Therapy, 19,* 547–549.

Fraser, D., Peterkin, G. S., Gamsu, C. V., & Baldwin, P. J. (1990). Benzodiazepine withdrawal: A pilot comparison of three methods. *British Journal of Clinical Psychology, 29,* 231–233.

Freedman, R. R., & Papsdorf, J. D. (1976). Biofeedback and progressive relaxation treatment of sleep-onset insomnia: A controlled, all night investigation. *Biofeedback and Self-Regulation, 1,* 253–271.

Freedman, R. R., & Sattler, H. L. (1982). Physiological and psychological factors in sleep-onset insomnia. *Journal of Abnormal Psychology, 91,* 380–389.

Freeman, A., Pretzer, J., Fleming, B., & Simon, K. M. (1990). *Clinical applications of cognitive therapy.* New York: Plenum Press.

Friedman, L., Bliwise, D. L., Yesavage, J. A., & Salom, S. R. (1991). A preliminary study comparing sleep restriction and relaxation treatments for insomnia in older adults. *Journal of Gerontology, 46,* P1–P8.

Gaillard, J. M. (1985). Neurochemical regulation of the states of alertness. *Annals of Clinical Research, 17,* 175–184.

Gallup Organization. (1979). *The Gallup study of sleeping habits.* Princeton, NJ: Author.

Gallup Organization. (1991). *Sleep in America.* Princeton, NJ: Author.

Garfield, S. L. (1989). *The practice of brief psychotherapy.* Elmsford, NY: Pergamon Press.

Gillin, J. C. (1983). The sleep therapies of depression. *Progress in Neuropsychopharmacology and Biological Psychiatry, 7,* 351–364.

Gillin, J. C., & Byerley, W. F. (1990). The diagnosis and management of insomnia. *New England Journal of Medicine, 322,* 239–248.

Gillin, J. C., Duncan, W., Pettigrew, K. D., Frankel, B. L., & Snyder, F. (1979). Successful separation of depressed, normal, and insomniac subjects by EEG sleep data. *Archives of General Psychiatry, 36,* 85–90.

Gillin, J. C., Spinweber, C. L., & Johnson, L. C. (1989). Rebound insomnia: A critical review. *Journal of Clinical Psychopharmacology, 9,* 161–172.

Gislason, T., & Almqvist, M. (1987). Somatic diseases and sleep complaints: An epidemiological study of 3201 Swedish men. *Acta Medica Scandinavica, 221,* 475–481.

Glovinsky, P. B., & Spielman, A. J. (1991). Sleep restriction therapy. In P. Hauri (Ed.), *Case studies in insomnia* (pp. 49–63). New York: Plenum Press.

Goldberg, H. L., & Finnerty, R. J. (1980). Trazodone in the treatment of neurotic depression. *Journal of Clinical Psychiatry, 41,* 430–434.

Good, R. (1975). Frontalis muscle tension and sleep latency. *Psychophysiology, 12,* 465–467.

Greenberg, G. D., Watson, R. K., & Deptula, D. (1987). Neuropsychological dysfunction in sleep apnea. *Sleep, 10,* 254–262.

Greenblatt, D. J. (1991). Benzodiazapine hypnotics: Sorting the pharmacokinetic facts. *Journal of Clinical Psychiatry, 52*(Suppl.), 4–10.

Greenblatt, D. J., Harmatz, J. S., Zinny, M. A., & Shader, R. I. (1987). Effect of gradual withdrawal on the rebound sleep disorder after discontinuation of triazolam. *New England Journal of Medicine, 317,* 722–728.

Greenblatt, D. J., & Shader, R. I. (1985). Clinical pharmacokinetics of the benzodiazepines. In D. E. Smith & D. R. Wesson (Eds.), *The benzodiazepines: Current standards for medical practice* (pp. 43–58). Lancaster, England: MTP Press.

Griffin, S. J., & Trinder, J. (1978). Physical fitness, exercise, and human sleep. *Psychophysiology, 5,* 447–450.

Gross, R. T., & Borkovec, T. D. (1982). Effects of cognitive intrusion manipulation on sleep-onset latency of good sleepers. *Behavior Therapy, 13,* 112–116.

Grosvenor, A., & Lack, L. C. (1984). The effect of sleep before or after learning on memory. *Sleep, 7,* 155–167.

Guilleminault, C. (1989). Clinical features and evaluation of obstructive sleep apnea. In M. H. Kryger, T. Roth, & W. C. Dement (Eds.), *Principles and practice of sleep medicine* (pp. 552–558). Philadelphia: Saunders.

Guilleminault, C., & Dement, W. C. (1977). Amnesia and disorders of excessive daytime sleepiness. In R. R. Drucker-Colin & J. L. McGaugh (Eds.), *Neurobiology of sleep and memory* (pp. 439–456). New York: Academic Press.

Hammond, E. C. (1964). Some preliminary findings on physical complaints from a prospective study of 1,064,004 men and women. *American Journal of Public Health, 54,* 11–23.

Hartmann, E. (1973). Sleep requirement: Long sleepers, short sleepers, variable sleepers, and insomniacs. *Psychosomatics, 14,* 95–103.

Hartmann, E. (1977). L-Tryptophan: A rational hypnotic with clinical potential. *American Journal of Psychiatry, 134,* 366–370.

Hauri, P. J. (1981). Treating psychophysiologic insomnia with biofeedback. *Archives of General Psychiatry, 38,* 752–758.

Hauri, P. J. (1982). *The sleep disorders.* Kalamazoo, MI: Upjohn.

Hauri, P. J. (1983). A cluster analysis of insomnia. *Sleep, 6,* 326–338.

Hauri, P. J. (Ed.). (1991). *Case studies in insomnia.* New York: Plenum Press.

Hauri, P. J., Chernik, D., Hawkins, D., & Mendels, J. (1974). Sleep of depressed patients in remission. *Archives of General Psychiatry, 31,* 386–391.

Hauri, P. J., & Fisher, J. (1986). Persistent psychophysiological (learned) insomnia. *Sleep, 9,* 38–53.

Hauri, P. J., Friedman, M., & Ravaris, C. L. (1989). Sleep in patients with spontaneous panic attacks. *Sleep, 12,* 323–337.

Hauri, P. J., & Olmstead, E. M. (1980). Childhood-onset insomnia. *Sleep, 3,* 59–65.

Hauri, P. J., & Olmstead, E. M. (1983). What is the moment of sleep onset for insomniacs? *Sleep, 6,* 10–15.

Hauri, P. J., & Olmstead, E. M. (1989). Reverse first night effect in insomnia. *Sleep, 12,* 97–105.

Hauri, P. J., Percy, L., Hellekson, C., Hartmann, E., & Russ, D. (1982). The treatment of psychophysiologic insomnia with biofeedback: A replication study. *Biofeedback and Self-Regulation, 7,* 223–235.

Hauri, P. J., & Silberfarb, P. M. (1980). Effects of aspirin on the sleep of insomniacs. *Current Therapeutic Research, 28,* 867–874.

Hauri, P. J., & Wisbey, J. (1992). Wrist actigraphy in insomnia. *Sleep, 15,* 293–301.

Haynes, S. N., Adams, A. E., & Franzen, M. (1981). The effects of presleep stress on sleep-onset insomnia. *Journal of Abnormal Psychology, 90,* 601–606.

Haynes, S. N., Adams, A. E., West, S., Kamens, L., & Safranek, R. (1982). The stimulus control paradigm in sleep-onset insomnia. *Journal of Psychosomatic Research, 26,* 333–339.

Haynes, S. N., Fitzgerald, S. G., Shute, G., & O'Meary, M. (1985). Responses of psychophysiologic and subjective insomniacs to auditory stimuli during sleep: A replication and extension. *Journal of Abnormal Psychology, 94,* 338–345.

Haynes, S. N., & O'Brien, W. H. (1990). Functional analysis in behavior therapy. *Clinical Psychology Review, 10,* 649–668.

Haynes, S. N., Sides, H., & Lockwood, G. (1977). Relaxation instructions and frontalis electromyographic feedback intervention with sleep-onset insomnia. *Behavior Therapy, 8,* 644–652.

Healy, E. S., Kales, A., Monroe, L. J., Bixler, E. O., Chamberlin, K., & Soldatos, C. R. (1981). Onset of insomnia: Role of life-stress events. *Psychosomatic Medicine, 43,* 439–451.

Heath, A. C., Kendler, K. S., Eaves, L. J., & Martin, N. G. (1990). Evidence for genetic influences on sleep disturbance and sleep pattern in twins. *Sleep, 13,* 318–335.

Hoch, C. C., Reynolds, C. F., Kupfer, D. J., Berman, S. R., Houck, P. R., & Stack, J. A. (1987). Self-report versus recorded sleep in healthy seniors. *Psychophysiology, 24,* 293–299.

Hoddes, E., Zarcone, V., Smythe, H., Phillips, R., & Dement, W. C. (1973). Quantification of sleepiness: A new approach. *Psychophysiology, 10,* 431–436.

Hoelscher, T. J., & Edinger, J. D. (1988). Treatment of sleep-maintenance insomnia in older adults: Sleep period reduction, sleep education, and modified stimulus control. *Psychology and Aging, 3,* 258–263.

Hoelscher, T. J., Erwin, C. W., Marsh, G. R., Webb, M. D., Radtke, R. A., & Lininger, A. L. (1987). Ambulatory sleep monitoring with the Oxford-Medilog 9000: Technical acceptability, patient acceptance and clinical indications. *Sleep, 10,* 606–607.

Hoelscher, T. J., Ware, J. C., & Bond, T. (1993, June). *Initial validation of the Insomnia Impact Scale.* Paper presented at the annual meeting of the American Sleep Disorders Association, Los Angeles.

Horne, J. A. (1978). A review of the biological effects of total sleep deprivation in man. *Biological Psychology, 7,* 55–102.

Horne, J. A. (1981). The effects of exercise upon sleep: A critical review. *Biological Psychology, 12,* 241–290.

Horne, J. A. (1985). Sleep function with particular reference to sleep deprivation. *Annals of Clinical Research, 17,* 199–208.

Horne, J. A. (1988a). Sleep loss and "divergent" thinking ability. *Sleep, 11,* 528–536.

Horne, J. A. (1988b). *Why we sleep: The functions of sleep in humans and other mammals.* Oxford: Oxford University Press.

Horne, J. A., & Staff, L. H. (1983). Exercise and sleep: body heating effects. *Sleep, 6,* 36–46.

Hughes, J. R., Higgins, S. T., Bickel, W. K., Hunt, W. K., Fenwick, J. W., Gulliver, S. B., & Mireault, G. C. (1991). Caffeine self-administration, withdrawal, and adverse effects among coffee drinkers. *Archives of General Psychiatry, 48,* 611–617.

Hughes, R. C., & Hughes, H. H. (1978). Insomnia: Effects of EMG biofeedback, relaxation training, and stimulus control. *Behavioral Engineering, 5,* 67–72.

Institute of Medicine. (1979). *Sleeping pills, insomnia, and medical practice.* Washington, DC: National Academy of Sciences.

Jacobs, E. A., Reynolds, C. F., Kupfer, D. J., Lovin, P. A., & Ehrenpreis, A. B. (1988). The role of polysomnography in the differential diagnosis of chronic insomnia. *American Journal of Psychiatry, 145,* 346–349.

Jacobs, G. D., Benson, H., & Friedman, R. (1993). Home-based central nervous system assessment of a multifactor behavioral intervention for chronic sleep-onset insomnia. *Behavior Therapy, 24,* 159–174.

Jacobs, G. D., Rosenberg, P., Friedman, R., Matheson, J., Peavy, G., Domar, & Benson, H. (in press). Multifactor behavioral treatment of chronic sleep-onset insomnia using stimulus control and the relaxation response: A preliminary study. *Behavior Modification.*

Johnson, L. C. (1982). Sleep deprivation and performance. In W. B. Webb (Ed.), *Biological rhythms, sleep, and performance* (pp. 111–141). New York: Wiley.

Johnson, L. C., Burdick, J. A., & Smith, J. (1970). Sleep during alcohol intake and withdrawal in the chronic alcoholic. *Archives of General Psychiatry, 22,* 406–418.

Johnson, L. C., & Chernik, D. A. (1982). Sedative–hypnotics and human performance. *Psychopharmacology, 76,* 101–113.

Jones, B. E. (1989). Basic mechanisms of sleep–wake states. In M. H. Kryger, T. Roth, & W. C. Dement (Eds.), *Principles and practice of sleep medicine* (pp. 121–138). Philadelphia: Saunders.

Kales, A., Bixler, E. O., Kales, J. D., & Scharf, M. B. (1977). Comparative effectiveness of nine hypnotic drugs: Sleep laboratory studies. *Journal of Clinical Pharmacology, 17,* 207–213.

Kales, A., Bixler, E. O., Soldatos, C. R., Vela-Mueno, A., Jacoby, J., & Kales, J. D. (1982). Quazepam and flurazepam: Long term use and withdrawal. *Clinical Pharmacology and Therapeutics, 32,* 781–788.

Kales, A., Bixler, E. O., Vela-Bueno, A., Cadieux, R. J., Soldatos, C. R., & Kales, J. D. (1984). Biopsychobehavioral correlates of insomnia: III. Polygraphic findings of sleep difficulty and their relationship to psychopathology. *International Journal of Neuroscience, 23,* 43–56.

Kales, A., Caldwell, A. B., Soldatos, C. R., Bixler, E. O., & Kales, J. D. (1983). Biopsychobehavioral correlates of insomnia: II. Pattern specificity and consistency with the MMPI. *Psychosomatic Medicine, 45,* 341–356.

Kales, A., & Kales, J. D. (1984). *Evaluation and treatment of insomnia.* New York: Oxford University Press.

Kales, A., Soldatos, C. R., Bixler, E. O., & Kales, J. D. (1983). Early morning insomnia with rapidly eliminated benzodiazepines. *Science, 220,* 95–97.

Kales, A., Soldatos, C. R., & Vela-Bueno, A. (1985). Clinical comparison of benzodiazepine hypnotics with short and long elimination half-lives. In D. E. Smith & D. R. Wesson (Eds.), *The benzodiazepines: Current standards for medical practice* (pp. 121–148). Lancaster, England: MTP Press.

Kales, A., & Vgontzas, A. N. (1992). Predisposition to and development and persistence of chronic insomnia: Importance of psychobehavioral factors [Editorial]. *Archives of Internal Medicine, 152,* 1570–1572.

Kales, J. D., Kales, A., Bixler, E. O., Soldatos, C. R., Cadieux, R. J., Kashurba, G. J., & Vela-Bueno, A. (1984). Biopsychobehavioral correlates of insomnia: V. Clinical characteristics and behavioral correlates. *American Journal of Psychiatry, 141,* 1371–1376.

Kales, J. D., Tan, T. L., Swearingen, C., & Kales, A. (1971). Are over-the-counter sleep medications effective? All-night EEG studies. *Current Therapeutic Research, 13,* 143–151.

Karacan, I., Thornby, J. I., Anch, A. M., Booth, G. H., Williams, R. L., & Salis, P. J. (1976). Dose related sleep disturbances induced by coffee and caffeine. *Clinical Pharmacology and Therapeutics, 20,* 682–689.

Kazarian, S. S., Howe, M. G., & Csapo, K. G. (1979). Development of the Sleep Behavior Self-Rating Scale. *Behavior Therapy, 10,* 412–417.

Kazdin, A. E. (1986). Comparative outcome studies in psychotherapy: Methodological issues and strategies. *Journal of Consulting and Clinical Psychology, 54,* 95–105.

King, D. A., Bouton, M. E., & Musty, R. E. (1987). Associative control of tolerance to the sedative effects of a short-acting benzodiazepine. *Behavioral Neuroscience, 101,* 104–114.

Kirmil-Gray, K., Eagleston, J. R., Thoresen, C. E., & Zarcone, V. P. (1985). Brief consultation and stress management treatments for drug-dependent insomnia: Effects on sleep quality, self-efficacy, and daytime stress. *Journal of Behavioral Medicine, 8,* 79–99.

Klink, M. E., Quan, S. F., Kaltenborn, W. T., & Lebowitz, M. D. (1992). Risk factors associated with complaints of insomnia in a general adult population: Influences of previous complaints of insomnia. *Archives of Internal Medicine, 152,* 1572–1575.

Kowatch, R. A. (1989). Sleep and head injury. *Psychiatric Medicine, 7,* 37–41.

Kramer, M., & Schoen, L. S. (1984). Problems in the use of long-acting hypnotics in older patients. *Journal of Clinical Psychiatry, 45,* 176–177.

Kripke, D. F., Simons, R. N., Garfinkel, L., & Hammond, E. C. (1979). Short and long sleep and sleeping pills: Is increased mortality associated? *Archives of General Psychiatry, 36,* 103–116.

Kryger, M. H., Steljes, D., Pouliot, Z., Neufeld, H., & Odynski, T. (1991). Subjective versus objective evaluation of hypnotic efficacy: Experience with zolpidem. *Sleep, 14,* 399–407.

Kuisk, L. A., Bertelson, A. D., & Walsh, J. K. (1989). Presleep cognitive hyperarousal and affect as factors in objective and subjective insomnia. *Perceptual and Motor Skills, 69,* 1219–1225.

Kwentus, J. A., Schultz, D. C., Fairman, P., & Isrow, L. (1985). Sleep apnea: A review. *Psychosomatics, 26,* 713–730.

Lacey, J. H., Crisp, A. H., Kalucy, R. S., Hartmann, M. K., & Chen, C. N. (1975). Weight gain and the sleeping electroencephalogram: Study of ten patients with anorexia nervosa. *British Medical Journal, iv,* 556–558.

Lacks, P. (1987). *Behavioral treatment of persistent insomnia.* Elmsford, NY: Pergamon Press.

Lacks, P. (1991). Stimulus control in a group setting. In P. J. Hauri (Ed.), *Case studies in insomnia* (pp. 29–47). New York: Plenum Press.

Lacks, P., Bertelson, A. D., Gans, L., & Kunkel, J. (1983). The effectiveness of three behavioral treatments for different degree of sleep-onset insomnia. *Behavior Therapy, 14,* 593–605.

Lacks, P., Bertelson, A. D., Sugerman, J., & Kunkel, J. (1983). The treatment of sleep-maintenance insomnia with stimulus control techniques. *Behaviour Research and Therapy, 21,* 291–295.

Lacks, P., & Morin, C. M. (1992). Recent advances in the assessment and treatment of insomnia. *Journal of Consulting and Clinical Psychology, 60,* 586–594.

Lacks, P., & Powlishta, K. (1989). Improvement following behavioral treatment for insomnia: Clinical significance, long-term maintenance, and predictors of outcome. *Behavior Therapy, 20,* 117–134.

Lacks, P., & Rotert, M. (1986). Knowledge and practice of sleep hygiene techniques in insomniacs and poor sleepers. *Behaviour Research and Therapy, 24,* 365–368.

Ladouceur, R., & Gros-Louis, Y. (1986). Paradoxical intention vs. stimulus control in the treatment of severe insomnia. *Journal of Behavior Therapy and Experimental Psychiatry, 17,* 267–269.

Levy, M., & Zylber-Katz, E. (1983). Caffeine metabolism and coffee-attributed sleep disturbances. *Clinical Pharmacology and Therapeutics, 6,* 770–775.

Libert, J. P., Bach, V., Johnson, L. C., Ehrhart, J., Wittersheim, & Keller, D. (1991). Relative and combined effects of heat and noise exposure on sleep in humans. *Sleep, 14,* 24–31.

Lichstein, K. L., & Fanning, J. (1990). Cognitive anxiety in insomnia: An analogue test. *Stress Medicine, 6,* 47–51.

Lichstein, K. L., & Fisher, S. M. (1985). Insomnia. In M. Hersen & A.S. Bellack (Eds.), *Handbook of clinical behavior therapy with adults* (pp. 319–352). New York: Plenum Press.

Lichstein, K. L., Hoelscher, T. J., Eakin, T. L., & Nickel, R. (1983). Empirical sleep assessment in the home: A convenient, inexpensive approach. *Journal of Behavioral Assessment, 5,* 111–118.

Lichstein, K. L., & Johnson, R. S. (1991). Older adults' objective self-recording of sleep in the home. *Behavior Therapy, 22,* 531–548.

Lichstein, K. L., & Johnson, R. S. (1993). Relaxation for insomnia and hypnotic use in older women. *Psychology and Aging, 8,* 103–111.

Lichstein, K. L., Johnson, R. S., Gupta, S. S., O'Laughlin, D. L., & Dykstra, T. A. (1992). Are insomniacs sleepy during the day? A pupillometric assessment. *Behaviour Research and Therapy, 30,* 283–292.

Lichstein, K. L., Nickel, R., Hoelscher, T. J., & Kelley, J. E. (1982). Clinical validation of a sleep assessment device. *Behaviour Research and Therapy, 20,* 292–297.

Lichstein, K. L., & Rosenthal, T. L. (1980). Insomniacs' perceptions of cognitive versus somatic determinants of sleep disturbance. *Journal of Abnormal Psychology, 89,* 105–107.

Lick, J., & Heffler, D. (1977). Relaxation training and attention placebo in the treatment of severe insomnia. *Journal of Consulting and Clinical Psychology, 45,* 153–161.

Liljenberg, B., Almqvist, M., Hetta, J., Roos, B. E., & Agren, H. (1989). Age and the prevalence of insomnia in adulthood. *European Journal of Psychiatry, 3,* 5–12.

Lozoff, B., Wolf, A. W., & Davis, N. S. (1985). Sleep problems seen in pediatric practice. *Pediatrics, 75,* 477–483.

Mamelak, M., Csima, A., & Price, V. (1984). A comparative 25-night sleep laboratory study on the effects of quazepam and triazolam on chronic insomniacs. *Journal of Clinical Pharmacology, 24,* 65–75.

Marchini, E. J., Coates, T. J., Magistad, J. G., & Waldum, S. J. (1983). What do insomniacs do, think, and feel during the day? A preliminary study. *Sleep, 6,* 147–155.

McCall, W. V., & Edinger, J. E. (1992). Subjective total insomnia: An example of sleep state misperception. *Sleep, 15,* 71–73.

McCall, W. V., Edinger, J. E., & Erwin, C. W. (1989). Clinical utility of casssette polysomnography in sleep and sleep-related disorders. In J. S. Ebersole (Ed.), *Ambulatory EEG monitoring* (pp. 267–275). New York: Raven Press.

McClusky, H. Y., Milby, J. B., Switzer, P. K., Williams, V., & Wooten, V. (1991). Efficacy of behavioral versus triazolam treatment in persistent sleep-onset insomnia. *American Journal of Psychiatry, 148,* 121–126.

McNair, D. M., Lorr, M., & Droppleman, L. F. (1971). *Manual for the Profile of Mood States.* San Diego, CA: Educational and Industrial Testing Service.

Meichenbaum, D. (1977). *Cognitive-behavior modification: An integrative approach.* New York: Plenum Press.

Meichenbaum, D. (1985). *Stress inoculation training.* Elmsford, NY: Pergamon Press.

Mellinger, G. D., Balter, M. B., & Uhlenhuth, E. H. (1985). Insomnia and its treatment: Prevalence and correlates. *Archives of General Psychiatry, 42,* 225–232.

Mellman, T. A., & Unde, T. W. (1989). Electroencephalographic sleep in panic disorder. *Archives of General Psychiatry, 46,* 178–184.

Mendelson, W. B. (1980). *The use and misuse of sleeping pills.* New York: Plenum Press.

Mendelson, W. B. (1987). *Human sleep: Research and clinical care.* New York: Plenum Press.

Miles, L. E., & Dement, W. C. (1980). Sleep and aging. *Sleep, 3,* 119–220.

Mindell, J. A. (1993). Sleep disorders in children. *Health Psychology, 12,* 152–163.

Mitchell, K. R. (1979). Behavioral treatment of presleep tension and intrusive cognitions in patients with severe predormital insomnia. *Journal of Behavioral Medicine, 2,* 57–69.

Mitchell, K. R., & White, R. G. (1977). Self-management of severe predormital insomnia. *Journal of Behavior Therapy and Experimental Psychiatry, 8,* 57–63.

Mitler, M. M., Carskadon, M. A., Czeisler, C. A., Dement, W. C., Dinges, D. F., & Graeber, R. C. (1988). Catastrophes, sleep, and public policy: Consensus report. *Sleep, 11,* 100–109.

Mitler, M. M., Carskadon, M. A., Phillips, R. L., Sterling, W. R., Zarcone, V. P., Spiegel, R., & Guilleminault, C. (1979). Hypnotic efficacy of temazepam: A long-term sleep laboratory evaluation. *British Journal of Clinical Pharmacology, 8,* 63–68.

Mitler, M. M., Poceta, S., Menn, S., & Erman, M. K. (1991). Insomnia in the chronically ill. In P.J. Hauri (Ed.), *Case studies in insomnia* (pp. 223–236). New York: Plenum Press.

Mitler, M. M., Seidel, W. F., Van Den Hoed, J., Greenblatt, D. J., & Dement, W. C. (1984). Comparative hypnotic effects of flurazepam, triazolam, and placebo: A long-term simultaneous nighttime and daytime study. *Journal of Clinical Psychopharmacology, 4,* 2–13.

Moldofsky, H. (1989). Sleep–wake mechanisms in fibrositis. *Journal of Rheumatology, 16*(Suppl.), 47–48.

Monk, T. H., Leng, V. C, Folkard, S., & Weitzman, E. D. (1983). Circadian rhythms in subjective alertness and core body temperature. *Chronobiologia, 10,* 49–55.

Monk, T. H., & Moline, M. L. (1989). The timing of bedtime and waketime decisions in free-running subjects. *Psychophysiology, 26,* 304–310.

Montplaisir, J., & Godbout, R. (1989). Restless legs syndrome and periodic movements during sleep. In M. Kryger, T. Roth, & W.C. Dement, (Eds), *Principles and practice of sleep medicine* (pp. 402–409). Philadelphia: Saunders.

Monroe, L. J. (1967). Psychological and physiological differences between good and poor sleepers. *Journal of Abnormal Psychology, 72,* 255–264.

Moran, M. G., Thompson, T. L., Nies, R., & Alan, S. (1988). Sleep disorders in the elderly. *American Journal of Psychiatry, 145,* 1369–1378.

Morawetz, D. (1989). Behavioral self-help treatment for insomnia: A controlled evaluation. *Behavior Therapy, 20,* 365–379.

Morgan, K., Dallosso, H., Ebrahim, S., Arie, T., & Fentem, P. H. (1988). Prevalence, frequency, and duration of hypnotic drug use among elderly living at home. *British Medical Journal, 296,* 601–602.

Morin, C. M. (1991). Approches cognitivo-comportementales dans le traitement de l'insomnie chronique. *Science et Comportement, 21,* 273–390.

Morin, C. M., & Azrin, N. H. (1985). *Social and clinical validation of insomnia treatment outcome.* Paper presented at the meeting of the Association for Advancement of Behavior Therapy, Houston.

Morin, C. M., & Azrin, N. H. (1987). Stimulus control and imagery training in treating sleep-maintenance insomnia. *Journal of Consulting and Clinical Psychology, 55,* 260–262.

Morin, C. M., & Azrin, N. H. (1988). Behavioral and cognitive treatments of geriatric insomnia. *Journal of Consulting and Clinical Psychology, 56,* 748–753.

Morin, C. M., Culbert, J. P., Kowatch, R. A., & Walton, E. (1989). Efficacy of cognitive-behavioral treatment for insomnia: A meta-analytic review. *Sleep Research, 18,* 272.

Morin, C. M., Culbert, J. P., & Schwartz, S. M. (1993). *Nonpharmacological interventions for insomnia: A meta-analysis of treatment efficacy.* Manuscript submitted for publication.

Morin, C. M., Gaulier, B., Barry, T., & Kowatch, R. A. (1992). Patients' acceptance of psychological and pharmacological therapies for insomnia. *Sleep, 15,* 302–305.

Morin, C. M., & Gramling, S. E. (1989). Sleep patterns and aging: Comparison of older adults with and without insomnia complaints. *Psychology and Aging, 4,* 290–294.

Morin, C. M., & Gramling, S. E. (1990). Sleep and chronic pain. In E. Catalano, *Getting to sleep* (pp. 159–185). Oakland, CA: New Harbinger Press.

Morin, C. M., Kowatch, R. A., Barry, T., & Walton, E. (1993). Cognitive-behavior therapy for late-life insomnia. *Journal of Consulting and Clinical Psychology, 61,* 137–146.

Morin, C. M., Kowatch, R. A., & O'Shanick, G. (1990). Sleep restriction for the inpatient treatment of insomnia. *Sleep, 13,* 183–186.

Morin, C. M., Kowatch, R. A., & Wade, J. (1989). Behavioral management of sleep disturbances secondary to chronic pain. *Journal of Behavior Therapy and Experimental Psychiatry, 20,* 295–302.

Morin, C. M., & Kwentus, J. A. (1988). Behavioral and pharmacological treatments for insomnia. *Annals of Behavioral Medicine, 10,* 91–100.

Morin, C. M., & Rapp, S. R. (1987). Behavioral management of geriatric insomnia. *Clinical Gerontologist, 4,* 15–24.

Morin, C. M., & Schoen, L. (1986). *Validation of an electromechanical timer to measure sleep/wake parameters.* Paper presented at the annual meeting of the Association for Advancement of Behavior Therapy, Chicago.

Morin, C. M., & Stone, J. (1992). *Cognitive management of dysfunctional beliefs and attitudes about sleep.* Paper presented at the World Congress of Cognitive Therapy, Toronto.

Morin, C. M., Stone, J., Maghakian, C., Astruc, M., Mercer, J., & Brink, D. (1993, June). *Cognitive-behavior therapy and pharmacotherapy for late-life insomnia: A placebo-controlled trial.* Paper presented at the annual meeting of the American Sleep Disorders Association, Los Angeles.

Morin, C. M., Stone, J., McDonald, K., & Jones, S. (1992). *Psychological management of insomnia: A clinical replication series with 100 patients.* Manuscript submitted for publication.

Morin, C. M., Stone, J., Trinkle, D., Mercer, J., & Remsberg, S. (in press). Dysfunctional beliefs and attitudes about sleep among older adults with and without insomnia complaints. *Psychology and Aging.*

Morris, M., Lack, L., & Dawson, D. (1990). Sleep-onset insomniacs have delayed temperature rhythms. *Sleep, 13,* 1–14.

Mullaney, D. J., Kripke, D. F., & Messin, S. (1980). Wrist-actigraphic estimation of sleep time. *Sleep, 3,* 83–92.

National Institutes of Health (NIH). (1984). Drugs and insomnia: The use of medications to promote sleep. *Journal of the American Medical Association, 18,* 2410–2414.

National Institutes of Health (NIH). (1991). Consensus Development Conference statement: The treatment of sleep disorders of older people. *Sleep, 14,* 169–177.

Nicassio, P. M., & Bootzin, R. R. (1974). A comparison of progressive relaxation and autogenic training as treatments for insomnia. *Journal of Abnormal Psychology, 83,* 253–260.

Nicassio, P. M., Boylan, M. B., & McCabe, T. G. (1982). Progressive relaxation, EMG biofeedback and biofeedback placebo in the treatment of sleep onset insomnia. *British Journal of Medical Psychology, 55,* 159–166.

Nicassio, P. M., Mendlowitz, D. R., Fussell, J. J., & Petras, L. (1985). The phenomenology of the pre-sleep state: The development of the Pre-Sleep Arousal Scale. *Behaviour Research and Therapy, 23,* 263–271.

Nicholson, A. N., Bradley, C. M., & Pasco, P. A. (1989). Medications: Effect on sleep and wakefulness. In M. H. Kryger, T. Roth, & W. C. Dement (Eds.), *Principles and practice of sleep medicine* (pp. 228–236). Philadelphia: Saunders.

Nicholson, A. N., & Stone, B. M. (1979a). L-Tryptophan and sleep in healthy men. *Electroencephalography and Clinical Neurophysiology, 47,* 539–545.

Nicholson, A. N., & Stone, B. M. (1979b). Diazepam and 3 hydroxydiazepam (temazepam) and sleep of middle age. *British Journal of Clinical Pharmacology, 7,* 463–468.

Nino-Murcia, G., & Dement, W. C. (1987). Psychophysiological and pharmacological aspects of somnambulism and night terrors in children. In H.Y. Meltzer (Ed.), *Psychopharmacology: The third generation of progress* (pp. 873–879). New York: Raven Press.

Ogilvie, R. D., & Wilkinson, R. T. (1984). The detection of sleep onset: Behavioral and physiological convergence. *Psychophysiology, 21,* 510–520.

Ogilvie, R. D., Wilkinson, R. T., & Allison, S. (1989). The detection of sleep onset: Behavioral, physiological, and subjective convergence. *Sleep, 12,* 458–474.

Orem, J., & Barnes, C. D. (1980). *Physiology in sleep.* New York: Academic Press.

Parkes, J.D. (1985). *Sleep and its disorders.* Philadelphia: Saunders.

Pierce, M. W., & Shu, V. S. (1990). Efficacy of estazolam. *American Journal of Medicine, 88*(Suppl.), 6–11.

Pilowsky, I., Crettenden, I., & Townley, M. (1985). Sleep disturbance in pain clinic patients. *Pain, 23,* 27–33.

Poling, A., Gadow, K. D., & Cleary, J. (1991). *Drug therapy for behavior disorders: An introduction.* Elmsford, NY: Pergamon Press.

Pollak, C. P., Perlick, D., Linsner, J. P., Wenston, J., & Hsieh, F. (1990). Sleep problems in the community elderly as predictors of death and nursing home placement. *Journal of Community Health, 15,* 123–135.

Pressman, M. R. (1991). Whatever happened to insomnia (and insomnia research)? [Editorial]. *American Journal of Psychiatry, 148,* 419–420.

Price, V. A., Coates, T. J., Thoresen, C. E., & Grinstead, O. A. (1978). Prevalence and correlates of poor sleep among adolescents. *American Journal of Diseases of Children, 132,* 583–586.

Prinz, P. N., Vitiello, M. V., Raskind, M. A., & Thorpy, M. J. (1990). Geriatrics: Sleep disorders and aging. *New England Journal of Medicine, 323,* 520–526.

Puder, R., Lacks, P., Bertelson, A. D., & Storandt, M. (1983). Short term stimulus control treatment of insomnia in older adults. *Behavior Therapy, 14,* 424–429.

Rechtschaffen, A., & Kales, A. (1968). *A manual of standardized terminology, techniques, and scoring system for sleep stages of human subjects.* Los Angeles: BIS/BRI, UCLA.

Regenstein, Q. R. (1980). Insomnia and sleep disturbances in the aged: Sleep and insomnia in the elderly. *Journal of Geriatric Psychiatry, 13,* 153–171.

Relinger, H., & Bornstein, P. H. (1979). Treatment of sleep onset insomnia by paradoxical intention. *Behavior Modification, 3,* 203–222.

Reynolds, C. F., & Kupfer, D. J. (1987). Sleep research in affective illness: State of the art circa 1987. *Sleep, 10,* 199–215.

Reynolds, C. F., Kupfer, D. J., Buysse, D. J., Coble, P., & Yeager, A. (1991). Subtyping DSM-III-R primary insomnia: A literature review by the DSM-IV Work Group on Sleep Disorders. *American Journal of Psychiatry, 148,* 432–438.

Reynolds, C. F., Kupfer, D. J., Taska, L. S., Hoch, C. C., Sewitch, D. W., & Spiker, D. G. (1985). The sleep of healthy seniors: A revisit. *Sleep, 8,* 20–29.

Reynolds, C. F., Shaw, D. M., Newton, T. F., Coble, P. A., & Kupfer, D. J. (1983). EEG sleep in outpatients with generalized anxiety: A preliminary comparison with depressed outpatients. *Psychiatric Research, 8,* 81–89.

Reynolds, C. F., Taska, L. S., Sewitch, D. E., Restifo, K., Coble, P. A., & Kupfer, D. J. (1984). Persistent psychophysiological insomnia: Preliminary research diagnostic criteria and EEG sleep data. *American Journal of Psychiatry, 141,* 804–805.

Richardson, G. S., Carskadon, M. A., Orav, E. J., & Dement, W. C. (1982). Circadian variation of sleep tendency in elderly and young adult subjects. *Sleep*, 5, S82–S94.

Rodin, J., McAvay, G., & Timko, C. (1988). A longitudinal study of depressed mood and sleep disturbances in elderly adults. *Journal of Gerontology*, 43, P45–P53.

Roehrs, T. A., Lamphere, J., Paxton, C., Wittig, R., Zorick, F., & Roth, T. (1984). Temazepam's efficacy in patients with sleep onset insomnia. *British Journal of Clinical Pharmacology*, 17, 691–696.

Roehrs, T. A., Tietz, E., Zorick, F., & Roth, T. (1984). Daytime sleepiness and antihistamines. *Sleep*, 7, 137–141.

Roehrs, T. A., Vogel, G., & Roth, T. (1990). Rebound insomnia: Its determinant and significance. *American Journal of Medicine*, 88(Suppl.), 39–42.

Roehrs, T. A., Zorick, F., Kaffeman, M., Sickelsteel, J., & Roth, T. (1982). Flurazepam for short-term treatment of complaint of insomnia. *Journal of Clinical Pharmacology*, 22, 290–296.

Roffward, H. P., Muzio, J. M., & Dement, W. C. (1966). Ontogenic development of the human sleep-dream cycle. *Science*, 152, 604–619.

Rosa, R., Bonnet, M. H., & Kramer, M. (1983). The relationship of sleep and anxiety in anxious subjects. *Biological Psychology*, 16, 119–126.

Rosen, R. C., & Kostis, J. B. (1985). Biobehavioral sequellae associated with adrenergic-inhibiting antihypertensive agents: A critical review. *Health Psychology*, 4, 579–604.

Rosenberg, R. (1991). Assessment and treatment of delayed sleep phase syndrome. In P. Hauri (Ed.), *Case studies in insomnia* (pp. 193–207). New York: Plenum Press.

Ross, R. J., Ball, W. A., Sullivan, K. A., & Caroff, S. N. (1989). Sleep disturbance as the hallmark of posttraumatic stress disorder. *American Journal of Psychiatry*, 146, 697–707.

Roth, T., Hartse, K., Saab, P. G., Piccione, P. M., & Kramer, M. (1980). The effects of flurazepam, lorazepam, and triazolam on sleep and memory. *Psychopharmacology*, 70, 231–237.

Roth, T., & Roehrs, T. A. (1991). A review of the safety profiles of benzodiazepine hypnotics. *Journal of Clinical Psychiatry*, 52(Suppl.), 38–41.

Roth, T., Zorick, F., Wittig, R., & Roehrs, T. A. (1982). Pharmacological and medical considerations in hypnotic use. *Sleep*, 5(Suppl.), 46–52.

Roy-Byrne, P. P., & Cowley, D. S. (Eds.). (1991). *Benzodiazepines in clinical practice: Risks and benefits*. Washington, DC: American Psychiatric Press.

Roy-Byrne, P. P., & Hommer, D. (1988). Benzodiazepine withdrawal: Overview and implications for the treatment of anxiety. *American Journal of Medicine*, 84, 1041–1051.

Rubinstein, M. L., Rothenberg, S.A., Maheswaran, S., Tsai, J. S., Zozula, R., & Spielman, A. J. (1990). Modified sleep restriction therapy in the middle-aged and elderly chronic insomniacs. *Sleep Research*, 19, 276.

Rubman, S., Brantley, P. J., Waters, W. F., Jones, G. N., Constans, J. I., & Findley, J.C. (1990). *Daily stress and insomnia*. Paper presented at the meeting of the Society of Behavioral Medicine, Chicago.

Rush, A. J., Erman, M. K., Giles, D. E., Schlesser, M. A., Carpenter, G., Vasavuda, N., & Roffward, H. P. (1986). Polysomnographic findings in recently drug-free and clinical remitted patients. *Archives of General Psychiatry*, 43, 878–884.

Salin-Pascual, R. J., Roehrs, T. A., Merlotti, L. A., Zorick, F., & Roth, T. (1992). Long-term study of the sleep of insomnia patients with sleep state misperception and other insomnia patients. *American Journal of Psychiatry*, 149, 904–908.

Sanchez-Craig, M., Kay, G., Busto, V., & Cappell, H. (1986). Cognitive-behavioural treatment for benzodiazepine dependence. *Lancet*, 8471, 388.

Sanford, I. R. (1975). Tolerance of debility in elderly dependents by supports at home: Its significance for hospital practice. *British Medical Journal*, 3, 471–473.

Sanavio, E. (1988). Pre-sleep cognitive intrusions and treatment of onset-insomnia. *Behaviour Research and Therapy, 26,* 451–459.

Sanavio, E., Vidotto, G., Bettinardi, O., Rolletto, T., & Zorzi, M. (1990). Behavior therapy for DIMS: Comparison of three treatment procedures with follow-up. *Behavioural Psychotherapy, 18,* 151–167.

Saskin, P., Moldofsky, H., & Lue, F. A. (1986). Sleep and posttraumatic rheumatic pain modulation disorder (fibrositis syndrome). *Psychosomatic Medicine, 48,* 319–323.

Schenck, C. H., Milner, D. M., Hurwitz, T. D., Bundlie, S. R., & Mahowald, M. W. (1989). A polysomnographic and clinical report on sleep-related injury in 100 adult patients. *American Journal of Psychiatry, 146,* 1166–1173.

Schneider-Helmert, D. (1985). Overestimation of hypnotic drug effects by insomniacs: A hypothesis. *Psychopharmacology, 87,* 107–110.

Schneider-Helmert, D. (1987). Twenty-four hour sleep–wake function and personality patterns in chronic insomniacs and healthy controls. *Sleep, 10,* 452–462.

Schneider-Helmert, D. (1988). Why low-dose benzodiazepine-dependent insomniacs can't escape their sleeping pills. *Acta Psychiatrica Scandinavica, 78,* 706–711.

Schoicket, S. L., Bertelson, A. D., & Lacks, P. (1988). Is sleep hygiene a sufficient treatment for sleep maintenace insomnia? *Behavior Therapy, 19,* 183–190.

Seidel, W. F., Ball, S., Cohen, S., Patterson, N., Yost, D., & Dement, W. C. (1984). Daytime alertness in relation to mood, performance, and nocturnal sleep in chronic insomniacs and noncomplaining sleepers. *Sleep, 7,* 230–258.

Sewitch, D. E. (1984). NREM sleep continuity and the sense of having slept in normal sleepers. *Sleep, 7,* 147–154.

Sewitch, D. E., & Kupfer, D. J. (1985). Polysomnographic telemetry using Telediagnostic and Oxford Medilog 9000 Systems. *Sleep, 8,* 288–293.

Shaffer, J. I., Dickel, M. J., Marik, N., & Slak, S. (1985). The effect of excessive motivation to fall asleep on sleep-onset. *Sleep Research, 14,* 102.

Shapiro, C. M., Bortz, R., Mitchell, D., Bartel, P., & Jooste, P. (1981). Slow-wave sleep: A recovery period after exercise. *Science, 214,* 1253–1254.

Shealy, R. C., Lowe, J., & Ritzler, B. (1980). Sleep onset insomnia: Personality characteristics and treatment outcome. *Journal of Consulting and Clinical Psychology, 48,* 659–661.

Shipley, J. E., Kupfer, D. J., Griffin, S. J., Dealy, R. S., Coble, P. A., McEachran, A. B., Grocho-Cinski, V. J., & Ulrich, R. F. (1985). Comparison of effects of desipramine and amitriptyline on EEG sleep of depressed patients. *Psychopharmacology, 85,* 14–25.

Shute, G. E., Fitzgerald, S. G., & Haynes, S. N. (1986). The relationship between internal attentional control and sleep-onset latency in older adults. *Journal of Gerontology, 41,* 770–773.

Siegel, S. (1983). Classical conditioning, drug tolerance, and drug dependence. In Y. Israel, F. B. Glaser, H. Kalant, R. E. Popham, W. Schmidt, & R. E. Smart (Eds.), *Research advances in alcohol and drug problems* (Vol. 7, pp. 207–246). New York: Plenum Press.

Smith, C., & Lapp, L. (1991). Increases in number of REMS and REM density in humans following an intensive learning period. *Sleep, 14,* 325–330.

Smith, M. L., Glass, G. V., & Miller, T. I. (1980). *The benefits of psychotherapy.* Baltimore: Johns Hopkins University Press.

Snyder, S., & Karacan, I. (1985). Sleep patterns of sober chronic alcoholics. *Neuropsychobiology, 13,* 97–100.

Soldatos, C. R., Kales, J. D., Scharf, M. B., Bixler, E. O., & Kales, A. (1980). Cigarette smoking associated with sleep difficulty. *Science, 207,* 551–553.

Spielberger, C. D., Gorsuch, R. L., & Lushene, R. E. (1970). *Manual for the State–Trait Anxiety Inventory.* Palo Alto, CA: Consulting Psychologists Press.

Spielman, A. J. (1986). Assessment of insomnia. *Clinical Psychology Review, 6,* 11–26.

Spielman, A. J., Caruso, L. S., & Glovinsky, P. B. (1987). A behavioral perspective on insomnia treatment. *Psychiatric Clinics of North America, 10,* 541–553.

Spielman, A. J., & Glovinsky, P. (1991). The varied nature of insomnia. In P. J. Hauri (Ed.), *Case studies in insomnia* (pp. 1–15). New York: Plenum Press.

Spielman, A. J., Saskin, P., & Thorpy, M. J. (1987). Treatment of chronic insomnia by restriction of time in bed. *Sleep, 10,* 45–56.

Spinweber, C. L., & Johnson, L. C. (1982). Effects of triazolam (0.5 mg) on sleep, performance, memory, and arousal threshold. *Psychopharmacology, 76,* 5–12.

Stanton, H. E. (1989). Hypnotic relaxation and the reduction of sleep onset insomnia. *International Journal of Psychosomatics, 36,* 64–68.

Stepanski, E. J., Koshorek, G., Zorick, F., Glinn, M., Roehrs, T. A., & Roth, T. (1989). Characteristics of individuals who do or do not seek treatment for chronic insomnia. *Psychosomatics, 30,* 421–427.

Stepanski, E. J., Zorick, F., Roehrs, T. A., Young, D., & Roth, T. (1988). Daytime alertness in patients with chronic insomnia compared with asymptomatic control subjects. *Sleep, 11,* 54–60.

Stone, J., Morin, C. M., Hart, R., Remsberg, S., & Mercer, J. (1992). *Neuropsychological functioning among older insomniacs with and without sleep apnea.* Manuscript submitted for publication.

Storms, M. D., & Nisbett, R. E. (1970). Insomnia and the attribution process. *Journal of Personality and Social Psychology, 16,* 319–328.

Sugerman, J. L., Stern, J. A., & Walsh, J. K. (1985). Daytime alertness in subjective and objective insomnia: Some preliminary findings. *Biological Psychiatry, 20,* 741–750.

Sweetwood, H., Grant, I., Kripke, D. F., Gerst, M. S., & Yager, J. (1980). Sleep disorder over time: Psychiatric correlates among males. *British Journal of Psychiatry, 136,* 456–462.

Tan, T. L., Kales, J. D., Kales, A., Martin, E. D., Mann, L. D., & Soldatos, C. R. (1987). Inpatient multidimensional management of treatment-resistant insomnia. *Psychosomatics, 28,* 266–272.

Tan, T. L., Kales, J. D., Kales, A., Soldatos, C. R., & Bixler, E. O. (1984). Biopsychobehavioral correlates of insomnia: IV. Diagnosis based on DSM-III. *American Journal of Psychiatry, 141,* 357–362.

Tokartz, T. P., & Lawrence, P. S. (1974). *An analysis of temporal and stimulus factors in the treatment of insomnia.* Paper presented at the meeting of the Association for Advancement of Behavior Therapy, Chicago.

Torsvall, L. (1981). Sleep after exercise: A literature review. *Journal of Sports Medicine, 21,* 218–225.

Trinder, J. (1988). Subjective insomnia without objective findings: A pseudo diagnostic classification? *Psychological Bulletin, 103,* 87–94.

Turk, D. C., Meichenbaum, D., & Genest, M. (1983). *Pain and behavioral medicine: A cognitive-behavioral perspective.* New York: Guilford Press.

Turner, R. M., & Ascher, L. M. (1979). Controlled comparison of progressive relaxation, stimulus control, and paradoxical intention therapies for insomnia. *Journal of Consulting and Clinical Psychology, 47,* 500–508.

Turner, R. M., & Ascher, L. M. (1982). Therapist factor in the treatment of insomnia. *Behaviour Research and Therapy, 20,* 33–40.

Turner, R. M., DiTomasso, R., & Giles, T. (1983). Failures in the treatment of insomnia: A plea for differential diagnosis. In E. B. Foa & P. M. G. Emmelkamp (Eds.), *Failures in behavior therapy* (pp. 284–304). New York: Wiley.

U.S. Public Health Service. (1976). *Physicians' drug prescribing patterns in skilled nursing facilities.* Washington, DC: U.S. Department of Health, Education and Welfare.

Van Egeren, L., Haynes, S. N., Franzen, M., & Hamilton, J. (1983). Presleep cognitions and attributions in sleep-onset insomnia. *Journal of Behavioral Medicine, 6,* 217–232.

Van Oot, P. H., Lane, T. W., & Borkovec, T. D. (1984). Sleep disturbances. In P. B. Sutker & H. Adams (Eds), *Handbook of psychopathology* (pp. 683–723). New York: Plenum Press.

Viens, M., De Koninck, J., Van Den Bergen, H., Audet, R., & Christ, G. (1988). A refined switch-activated time monitor for the measurement of sleep-onset latency. *Behaviour Research and Therapy, 26,* 271–273.

Vogel, G. W., Scharf, M., Walsh, J. K., & Roth, T. (1989). Effect of chronically administered zolpidem on the sleep of healthy insomniacs. *Sleep Research, 18,* 90.

Walsh, J. K., & Sugerman, J. L. (1989). Disorders of initiating and maintaining sleep in adult psychiatric disorders. In M. H. Kryger, T. Roth, & W. C. Dement (Eds.), *Principles and practices of sleep medicine* (pp. 448–455).Philadelphia: Saunders.

Ware, J. C. (1983). Tricyclic antidepressants in the treatment of insomnia. *Journal of Clinical Psychiatry, 44,* 25–28.

Ware, J. C. (1987). Evaluation of impotence: Monitoring periodic penile erections during sleep. *Psychiatric Clinics of North America, 10,* 675–686.

Ware, J. C., Brown, F. W., Moorad, P. J., Pitlard, J. T., & Cobert, B. (1989). Effects on sleep: A double-blind study comparing trimipramine and imipramine in depressed insomniac patients. *Sleep, 12,* 537–549.

Waters, W. F., Adams, S., Binks, P., & Varnado, P. (1993). Attention, stress, and negative emotion in persistent sleep-onset and sleep-maintenance insomnia. *Sleep, 16,* 128–136.

Webb, W. B. (1979). Theories of sleep functions and some clinical applications. In R. Drucker-Colin, M. Shkurovich, & M.B. Sterman (Eds.), *The function of sleep* (pp. 19–35). New York: Academic Press.

Webb, W. B. (1988). An objective behavioral model of sleep. *Sleep, 11,* 488–496.

Webb, W. B. (1989). Age-related changes in sleep. *Clinical Geriatric Medicine, 5,* 275–287.

Webb, W. B., & Agnew, H. W. (1971). Stage 4 sleep: Influence of time course variables. *Science, 174,* 1354–1356.

Webb, W. B., & Agnew, H. W. (1974). The effects of chronic limitation of sleep length. *Psychophysiology, 11,* 265–274.

Webb, W. B., & Agnew, H. W. (1975). Sleep efficiency for sleep-wake cycles of varied length. *Psychophysiology, 12,* 637–641.

Webb, W. B., Bonnet, M., & Blume, G. (1976). A post-sleep inventory. *Perceptual and Motor Skills, 43,* 987–993.

Webb, W. B., & Campbell, S. S. (1980). Awakenings and the return to sleep in an older population. *Sleep, 3,* 41–46.

Webb, W. B., & Levy, C. M. (1982). Age, sleep deprivation, and performance. *Psychophysiology, 19,* 272–276.

Weitzman, E. D., Czeisler, C. A., Coleman, R. M., Spielman, A. J., Zimmerman, J. C., Dement, W. C., Richardson, G. S., & Pollack, C. P. (1981). Delayed sleep phase syndrome: A chronobiologic disorder with sleep onset insomnia. *Archives of General Psychiatry, 38,* 737–746.

Weitzman, E. D., Czeisler, C. A., Zimmerman, J. C., Ronda, J. M., & Knauer, R. S. (1982). Chronobiological disorders: Analytic and therapeutic techniques. In C. Guillemninault (Ed.), *Sleeping and waking disorders: Indications and techniques* (pp. 297–329). Menlo Park, CA: Addison-Wesley.

Wever, R. (1979). *The circadian system of man: Results of experiments under temporal isolation.* New York: Springer-Verlag.

White, B., & Sanders, S. H. (1985). Differential effects on pain and mood in chronic pain patients with time- versus pain-contingent medication delivery. *Behavior Therapy, 16,* 28–38.

White, J. L., & Nicassio, P. M. (1990, November). *The relationship between daily stress, pre-sleep arousal, and sleep disturbance in good and poor sleepers.* Paper presented at the meeting of the Association for Advancement of Behavior Therapy, San Francisco.

Williams, R. L. (1988). Sleep disturbances in various medical and surgical conditions. In R. L. Williams, I. Karacan, & C. A. Moore (Eds.), *Sleep disorders: Diagnosis and treatment* (pp. 265–291). New York: Wiley.

Williams, R. L., Karacan, I., & Hursch, C. J. (1974). *EEG of human sleep: Clinical applications.* New York: Wiley.

Wittig, R. M., Zorick, F. J., Blumer, D., Heilbroon, M., & Roth, T. (1982). Disturbed sleep in patients complaining of chronic pain. *Journal of Nervous and Mental Disease, 170,* 429–431.

Wolfson, A., Lacks, P., & Futterman, A. (1992). Effects of parent training on infant sleeping patterns, parents' stress, and perceived parental competence. *Journal of Consulting and Clinical Psychology, 60,* 41–48.

Woolfolk, R. L., Kaffashan, L., & McNulty, T. F. (1976). Meditation training as treatment for insomnia. *Behavior Therapy, 7,* 359–365.

Woolfolk, R. L., & McNulty, T. F. (1983). Relaxation treatment for insomnia: A component analysis. *Journal of Consulting and Clinical Psychology, 51,* 495–503.

Wooten, V. (1989). Medical causes of insomnia. In M. H. Kryger, T. Roth, & W. C. Dement (Eds.), *Principles and practice of sleep medicine,* (pp. 456–475). Philadelphia: Saunders.

World Health Organization. (1993). *International classification of diseases* (10th ed.). Geneva: Author.

Zammit, G. K. (1988). Subjective ratings of the characteristics and sequelae of good and poor sleep in normals. *Journal of Clinical Psychology, 44,* 123–130.

Zarcone, V. P. (1989). Sleep hygiene. In M. Kryger, T. Roth, & W. Dement (Eds.), *Principles and practice of sleep medicine* (pp. 490–493). Philadelphia: Saunders.

Zorick, F. J., Roth, T., Hartse, K. M., Piccione, P., & Stepanski, E. (1981). Evaluation and diagnosis of persistent insomnia. *American Journal of Psychiatry, 138,* 769–773.

Zwart, C. A., & Lisman, S. A. (1979). Analysis of stimulus control treatment of sleep-onset insomnia. *Journal of Consulting and Clinical Psychology, 47,* 113–118.

# Index